Sexuality and Fertility after Cancer

Leslie R. Schover, Ph.D.

John Wiley & Sons, Inc.

New York • Chichester • Weinheim • Brisbane • Singapore • Toronto

To my friend and colleague, Dr. Wendy Schain, whose voice and example have guided me and helped so many women and men find joy in life after cancer.

Copyright © 1997 by Leslie Schover
Illustrations © 1997 by the Cleveland Clinic Foundation

Published by John Wiley & Sons, Inc.

Library of Congress Cataloging-in-Publication Data

Schover, Leslie R.
    Sexuality and fertility after cancer / Leslie Schover.
      p. cm.
    Includes bibliographical references and index.
    ISBN 0-471-18194-3 (pbk. : alk. paper)
    1. Cancer—Patients—Sexual behavior. 2. Fertility. 3. Cancer—
Complications. 4. Sex (Psychology) 5. Cancer—Surgery—
Complications. I. Title.
    [DNLM: 1. Neoplasms—psychology—popular works. 2. Sex Behavior—
psychology—popular works. 3. Sex Disorders—popular works.
4. Infertility—popular works. 5. Attitude to Health—popular
works.   QZ 201 S376a 1997]
RC262.S436 1997
616.99'4—dc21

Printed in the United States of America

10 9 8 7 6 5 4 3 2 1

Contents

PART II   IS THERE A PROBLEM? WHY IT HAPPENED AND HOW TO FIX IT

PART III FERTILITY AND PREGNANCY: WHEN CANCER ADDS INSULT TO INJURY

PART IV   SPECIAL STROKES FOR SPECIAL FOLKS

Acknowledgments

This book is the culmination of the most important aspect of my career—my clinical work and research on sexual problems and infertility after cancer treatment. Because sexuality is such a private area, the vignettes you will read in this book are composites based on my years of experience, rather than on actual accounts of patients I have known. I want to take this opportunity, however, to thank all the men and women who trusted me over the years with their most intimate stories. I hope that by summarizing all that I have learned, I can give something back to the community of cancer survivors to equal the gift of knowledge and inspiration that I have received.

I also want to thank some very special colleagues. First and foremost are the two Andys: Andrew von Eschenbach, M.D., Chairman of the Department of Urology at the University of Texas M. D. Anderson Cancer Center, and Andrew Novick, M.D., Chairman of the Department of Urology at the Cleveland Clinic Foundation. It was Andy von Eschenbach who began the program of sexual rehabilitation at M. D. Anderson and introduced me to this whole topic area. He has been an important role model and source of encouragement ever since. Andy Novick has unflaggingly supported my work in his department for the past ten years and has provided a stimulating and nurturing place to work. I have been extremely lucky to work with two premier surgeons who put such a high priority on patients' quality of life. I would also like to thank Maury Markman, M.D., Director of the Cleveland Clinic's Cancer Center, for his support of my efforts.

I would also like to acknowledge several other friends and colleagues whose advice and support have been especially important to me over the years: Joseph LoPiccolo, Ph.D., Wendy Schain, Ed.D., and David Wellisch, Ph.D. During the course of working on this book, I have had two excellent editors at John Wiley & Sons: PJ Dempsey, who had faith in the first draft and helped me make it into a trade book, and Judith McCarthy, who guided the production phase. I also thank my agent, Sidney Kramer, for his guidance.

Finally, I thank my family for their patience during the writing process: my husband, Menachem, whose optimism helps me stop catastrophizing; my son, Oren, who gave up some of our precious time together; and my father, Donald, who thinks everything I write is wonderful.

Introduction

Sex and *cancer* are two words that do not seem to belong in the same sentence. We think of sexuality as a force for joy and new life, whereas cancer is a death force. Increasingly, however, men and women survive their cancers. In the United States today, 8 million people have had cancer—with 5 million of them alive for more than five years since their diagnosis. Being able to enjoy sex is one important battle in winning the war against cancer.

Unfortunately, many types of cancer treatment physically damage men's and women's sexual functioning and fertility. Sexual problems are especially likely after cancers of the breast and prostate, the most common types of cancer in women and in men, respectively. The emotional stress of cancer also can create difficulties in sexual relationships. However, a variety of psychological and medical treatments are available to restore sexual function. Most people do not need months of psychotherapy or medical treatment to recover satisfying sex lives after cancer treatment. Rather they require some accurate information on what to expect and how to make the most of the available options for help. New treatments for infertility also open up possibilities for younger men and women who have survived cancer.

This book offers information to help you or a loved one to enjoy sex and to make informed choices about pregnancy in spite of cancer treatment. I wrote it because in fifteen years as a psychologist working with cancer patients, I saw that reproductive health problems rarely get discussed or treated in medical settings. Doctors and nurses are typically too busy and overwhelmed to take time to ask about patients' sex lives. Often they feel embarrassed discussing sex or do not have the knowledge to answer questions or to steer patients to someone who can give them the help they need. The impact of cancer treatment on fertility is also rarely explained fully. At major cancer centers, patients sometimes are actually offered special counseling. For patients who see a doctor in a smaller hospital, however, and especially for those who live in a rural area, help for a sexual or fertility problem is hardly ever made available. A book cannot substitute for good health care, but it can provide accurate information on the causes and treatments of these problems after cancer, present some techniques to try at home, and suggest how to find more help in your local community.

The Importance of Sexuality and Fertility

"Why is he worrying about sex? He should be glad he's still alive after having cancer." I have heard this comment a hundred times, in one form or another. Sometimes it is made by a doctor or sometimes by a patient's spouse. Occasionally, it is even an apology made by a man or woman who has survived cancer: "I know I should be grateful to be alive, but . . ."

Although our society has overemphasized sex in recent years, it is undeniably important. It is not only the way we reproduce ourselves, but also a basic element of relationship happiness. One study found that men's or women's ratings of their marital satisfaction could be predicted by adding up how often they had sex and subtracting the number of times they had arguments. Sex is the grease on the wheels of marriage. It helps couples smooth out the everyday tensions and disagreements they face. The majority of Americans stay sexually active, even in their older years. Although sexual pleasure may not be your top priority, the loss of the capacity to enjoy sex can be very sad.

Of course some men or women frankly could care less about staying sexually active after cancer treatment. They may have given up sex long ago, so one more handicap is not an issue. For those who never enjoyed sex much, cancer treatment may offer welcome permission to say "no" to sex.

Infertility is an issue for many survivors of childhood cancers and for younger men and women who undergo cancer treatment as adults. Cancer treatments not only can interfere with the physical ability to have sexual intercourse, but also can damage testicles, ovaries, and other parts of the reproductive system. Infertility and sexuality are linked. If a couple cannot have intercourse because of erection problems or a woman's vaginal pain, it will be difficult to conceive a child. If infertility is a source of emotional anguish, a couple may have a hard time getting in the mood for sex, even if they have no sexual problem per se. Thus sex remains a crucial part of quality of life after cancer.

Sexual Activity and Health

Two opposing views of sex are common. One is that sex is sinful and unhealthy, so celibacy would be the most healthy lifestyle. According to this philosophy, giving up sex would be the best choice after having cancer. The other viewpoint is that sex is necessary for health. If you take this view, resuming sex may help men and women live longer after a cancer diagnosis.

Which perspective is correct? From a scientific standpoint, neither one. There is no evidence that sexual activity interferes with health, unless you catch a sexually transmitted disease. Sex also is not necessary for good health. Each person has to make individual choices about whether it is worthwhile to pursue medical treatments or counseling or to make changes in a sexual routine in order to stay sexually active after cancer treatment.

Sexuality and the Stages of Your Life

Sex has different meanings for people of different ages. For teenagers, exploring sexual feelings is part of growing up. Issues of feeling attractive, developing healthy relationships, and learning how to experience sexual pleasure are foremost. For young adults, establishing more committed relationships and making decisions about pregnancy are major themes. As men and women age, sexuality loses its reproductive purpose but remains a vital part of intimacy. Needs for touch, emotional closeness, and physical pleasure do not decrease in later years. Sex is rated as an important ingredient both in long-term marriages and in new relationships that start after partners are widowed or divorced in older age.

This book will try to highlight issues important to both older and younger cancer survivors. Because cancer becomes more common with age, many readers of this book are probably over 50. The impact of aging on normal sexual function will be discussed in order to put the effects of cancer treatments for older men and women in the right context. Younger readers will not be neglected, however. It is often the men and women under age 50 who suffer most when cancer causes sexual problems. Books and pamphlets often fail to address the special concerns of childhood cancer survivors and those who face cancer earlier in adult life. The mechanics of sexual problems are similar across the boundaries of age, but emotional aspects of sex, fertility issues, and case examples will be discussed with specific age groups in mind.

Stages of Cancer Treatment and Your Sex Life

Some readers may just have found out about their cancer and face decisions about cancer treatment. Others are in the midst of their treatment or have finished it recently. Many readers are already long-term cancer survivors. The types of questions you have about sex may differ depending on your place on the time line of cancer treatment.

At the time of cancer diagnosis, sheer life or death is usually your highest priority, but as the medical team proposes treatments, you may start worrying about losing sexual function or attractiveness. Such decisions as whether to have a mastectomy or lumpectomy, to undergo pelvic radiation or radical prostatectomy for prostate cancer, to bank sperm, or to have your ovaries removed often rest in part on your own priorities. Even more commonly, you may not discuss sex at all with doctors or nurses until after treatment is over. As other aspects of life return to normal, a continuing sexual problem becomes more upsetting. Even then, many people do not seek help. In counseling cancer patients, I often see problems that have persisted for two, or four, or even ten years after treatment, problems that could have been solved long before. It is rarely too late to improve matters when it comes to sex, but the window of opportunity to prevent or treat infertility is often much smaller.

It is my hope that this book will be useful to any man or woman with questions about cancer and sexuality. It presents a good deal of factual information that is not easily available to most cancer patients. Even if it does not answer your specific questions or give you useful ideas for staying sexually active, it should guide you in seeking professional help for a sexuality or infertility problem.

How to Use This Book

Whether you have had cancer or you have a loved one who has gone through cancer treatment, you are probably wondering whether this book will answer your unique questions and concerns. I have organized this book by focusing on needs and problems.

If you are wondering what is normal sexually after cancer treatment, read Part I: There *Is* Sex after Cancer! Chapters discuss cancer's impact on your emotions about sex, the normal sexual response in men and women, and ways to use both talk and action to get sexually active again after cancer.

If you have a particular sexual problem, you can find information about it in Part II: Is There a Problem? Why It Happened and How to Fix It. Chapters focus on how to find expert help for treating the most common problems after cancer: loss of desire for sex, erection problems, changes in pleasure or orgasm, and painful sex.

If you are concerned about infertility, read Part III: Fertility and Pregnancy: When Cancer Adds Insult to Injury. Chapters discuss how to find expert help, how cancer treatment causes infertility and the available treatment options, the safety of pregnancy after cancer, the health of children born to cancer survivors, and using third-party reproductive techniques.

People who have had breast or prostate cancer treatment, have had a radical cancer surgery, have survived a cancer in childhood, are gay, or are single will find their special needs addressed in Part IV: Special Strokes for Special Folks.

The Resources section gives you lists of recommended books, audio-tapes, videotapes, products to enhance sex, and useful organizations. If you want to look up the sources for information provided in the chapters, refer to the Bibliography at the end of the book. If you see a medical term that is unfamiliar, you can look it up in the Glossary.

Sexual Beliefs and Values

The United States is made up of many ethnic and religious cultural groups, each with its own views on sexuality. This book tries to be sensitive to minority Americans, who typically grow up with more conservative values on sex. Americans of African, Asian, or Hispanic origin often find it even more difficult than mainstream white Americans to discuss sex or to ask for help with a sexual problem.

Another type of sexual diversity is sexual orientation—whether someone falls in love and has relationships with people of the same or opposite sex. I think that homosexual desires are a biological force, not a moral choice. Gay men and women account for somewhere between 2 and 10 percent of Americans. They also can have cancer and need information about sex and fertility after their treatment. Chapter 27 focuses on some of their special concerns. It is difficult to use language throughout a book that would be right for a gay couple as well as a heterosexual couple. I try to use *partner* rather than *spouse* (also because many heterosexual encounters take place between partners who are not married) and to emphasize that for all couples, sex that involves penetration is just one type of erotic pleasure.

PART I

THERE *IS* SEX
AFTER CANCER!

1

Sex, Cancer, and Your Emotions

Although many cancer treatments interfere with sex physically, it is the emotional reactions people have to cancer that most commonly cause sexual problems.

Diagnosis: The Crisis of Survival

A diagnosis of cancer may come suddenly, as an unexpected finding during a routine checkup, or it may come after days or weeks of dread, for example, after finding a hard breast lump and going through a mammogram and biopsy. Whatever the process of discovering cancer, hearing the word *cancer* brings up fears of disability and death. For many people, sexuality is not even on the list of priorities at the time of diagnosis.

Fred was 72 when his family doctor found a lump on his prostate. Blood tests, prostate biopsies, and bone scans confirmed that Fred had prostate cancer and that it had already spread to his pelvis and spine. The doctors agreed that Fred should have hormone therapy. He was given a choice of having his testicles surgically removed or of taking a monthly hormone shot that would shut down his body's production of male hormones. Fred was warned that, either way, he was likely to lose most of his interest in sex and to have trouble having erections.

Fred's wife, Rose, had been suffering from heart failure on and off for the past five years. Her health was so fragile that their sex life had long ago dwindled to nothing. Fred chose surgery just because it would be more convenient than going to the doctor every month for a shot. He had little concern over the impact of losing his sex drive, but he was very worried about not being healthy enough to take care of Rose.

Sometimes, however, avoiding a loss of sexual function can be one of the highest priorities in choosing a cancer treatment.

Dan was also 72 when his prostate cancer was found with the new prostate specific antigen (PSA) blood test. Luckily, Dan's tumor was quite small and of a slow-growing cell type. Dan's doctors told him his options: He could have a radical prostatectomy, an operation that would remove the prostate and nearby glands and leave him with a high chance of erection problems. He could have radiation therapy, resulting in a 25-to-50-percent chance of erection problems. Or he could wait and have no treatment, with frequent checkups to make sure the cancer was not advancing.

Dan had been widowed at age 65, after a long-term marriage with a wife who never enjoyed sex much. When he retired, however, he got involved in volunteer work at his local hospital and met and married a divorced woman in her early fifties. When Dan's cancer was diagnosed, they had just had their fourth wedding anniversary. Because Dan was in excellent health aside from his prostate cancer, he and his wife had enjoyed a sexual renewal that had amazed them both. After reading that many prostate cancers discovered with PSA in older men were not life threatening, Dan opted for watchful waiting, postponing treatment unless it appeared that his cancer was starting to grow.

Sometimes the fear that cancer treatment could damage sexual attractiveness or function leads to tragic delays in diagnosis or to failures to have lifesaving treatments.

Rosita was told at age 45 that she had colon cancer. She had watched her father die of colon cancer and vividly remembered helping him take care of his colostomy. Rosita's surgeon told her that rectum-sparing surgery might be possible, given the location of her tumor. Rosita's two children were grown, and she was divorced and working. Her real pleasure in life was ballroom dancing, and she competed regularly with her partner in local dance contests. Even the possibility of a colostomy was more than she could endure. Rosita heard of a clinic in Mexico offering a new miracle anticancer serum. She took her life savings and went there for a two-month stay. She felt fine for a year after treatment in Mexico, but then her symptoms reappeared. Diagnostic tests showed that the cancer had advanced. It was too late for a curative treatment. Rosita had traded quality of life for survival.

Getting through Cancer Treatment

The physical and emotional discomforts of cancer treatment often interfere with staying sexually active. After cancer surgery, there typically is a healing period during which sex is not recommended. Most types of radiation therapy stretch over several weeks. Toward the end of treatment, local irritation in the target area of the radiation can be painful. Depending on the location of the radiation, nausea or urinary and bowel irritation can be temporary annoyances. Chemotherapy drugs all have unpleasant side effects. The degree to which normal life is possible depends on the types and doses of the drugs used, as well as on a person's individual response. Bone marrow transplants are often followed by several months of feeling fatigued or ill before energy levels begin to return to normal.

The desire for sex can be a strong force, however, and some people manage to keep their sex lives going.

> Kevin was in the hospital for several days at a time during his chemotherapy for testicular cancer. At age 19, his illness interrupted college and the dating relationship he had developed. His girlfriend, Angela, came to visit him whenever she could drive up for the weekend. During one hospital stay, a nurse walked in on Kevin and Angela kissing and caressing. "Get off his bed!" she scolded Angela. "Don't you know he could get an infection?" Kevin was so angry he threatened to leave the hospital. His oncologist intervened and told the nurse that she had overreacted. He also reassured Angela that sexual activity was not harmful to Kevin's health.

When Treatment Is Over

The end of cancer treatment can leave patients feeling let down, even though they had been longing for the final day. The miseries of treatment actually provide reassurance that the cancer is under attack. After treatment, patients face the waiting game, wondering if the cancer was really cured or if it will return. Anxiety about cancer often shoots up when it is time to go back to the doctor for a follow-up visit. Even when everything checks out okay, aches and pains or minor illnesses can evoke panic. Another reason for hitting emotional bottom when treatment is over is that it is safer. During treatment, patients muster their energy to endure pain, nausea, fatigue, or other side effects. After treatment, they are left feeling drained, with the uncertainties of the future, sometimes including fears about losing health insurance, employability, fertility, or important relationships. Getting back to normal may seem like a mountainous task.

Resuming your sex life is one way of feeling more whole and healthy again; but if you are depressed, fatigued, or feeling unattractive, you may be afraid to risk initiating sex, perhaps being rejected by your partner or finding that you are unable to function well.

It was Hal's wife, Janice, who brought up sex when they saw the doctor six months after he had finished chemotherapy for lymphoma. She asked if the chemotherapy was responsible for the fact that Hal had not even tried to have sex for over a year. Hal was surprised by his wife's question and protested that he still felt attracted to her.

The doctor offered a blood test to check Hal's sex hormones but said that chemotherapy rarely affected them. He asked Hal about his ability to get erections. Not only was Hal waking up in the mornings with good erections, but he had "experimented" with masturbation recently and found he could have good sexual arousal and reach orgasm. Hal confessed that he had felt nervous to try sex again with Janice and that the longer they went without sex, the harder it was to get started.

"Well, I miss our sex life," Janice told him a little tearfully, "but even more, I miss feeling close to you." When Janice and Hal went home, they talked more about the problem and ended up in bed. Although the frequency of sex in their life never quite returned to the level it had been before Hal's cancer, they soon were enjoying lovemaking again.

For many couples, the talk about resuming sex never occurs, and a problem might drag on for years.

Betsy thought that having breast reconstruction after her mastectomy would be all the help she needed in keeping her sex life normal. She did not bargain for the impact of having to stop taking estrogen. At age 59, Betsy was ten years past her menopause, but she had never suffered from hot flashes or vaginal dryness because she had been taking hormones. Without the hormones, she found that intercourse was painful. Penetration felt dry and tight, and she became really scared when she spotted blood afterward. Although she knew that vaginal bleeding could be a symptom of cancer, she felt ashamed as an unmarried woman to ask her gynecologist about it. Betsy and her boyfriend eventually broke up. Sexual frustration was a major factor.

Betsy did not date for three years, until she met an attractive widower in her Sunday school class. She told him about her breast cancer and even about her sexual problem. Betsy switched to a younger, female gynecologist, who explained that postmenopausal vaginal dryness had caused the bleeding after intercourse and gave her vaginal moisturizers and water-based lubricants. When Betsy and her new partner finally tried intercourse, they had spent a good deal of time on foreplay and used quite a bit of lubricant. Betsy was delighted to find that she had no pain.

Common Myths about Sex and Cancer

Sometimes men and women do not resume sex after cancer treatment because they believe in one or more of these common myths about a link between sex and cancer.

Myth #1: Sex Makes Cancer Grow

One such belief is that having sex causes cancer to grow or spread. No scientific study has ever suggested that sexual activity spurs the growth of cancer, even cancer of the breast or prostate.

Myth #2: Sex Causes Cancer

Sometimes people believe that their cancer was actually caused by a past sexual act or habit. Guilt about a common sexual behavior—sex outside of marriage, masturbation, oral sex—translates into self-blame for cancer. Some men or women even view their cancer as a divine punishment for past sexual sins. Most clergy agree that illness is not handed out from above as part of a heavenly sentencing program. If it were, why would so many loving and good people get cancer, while so many truly evil people live to a ripe and healthy old age? If patients view cancer as a punishment, they should talk to someone whose religious views they respect. Carrying a burden of guilt is not helpful when coping with a life-threatening illness.

Myth #3: Giving Up Sex Will Help Cure Cancer

Because sex is viewed as an unhealthy sort of pleasure by many people, some men and women see celibacy as a sort of sacrifice they can make to ensure a healthy future. If this is really part of their spiritual beliefs, so be it. It might be worth it for them to reexamine the idea, however, to see if it is based more on superstition than on theology. There is certainly no scientific evidence that celibacy improves physical health.

Myth #4: Cancer Is Contagious Through Sex

Cancer is not a sexually transmitted disease. A cancer cell from one person's body cannot be successfully transplanted to a second person's body. The second person's immune system would recognize it as a stranger and kill it off. Confusion sometimes results from news stories about transplanting tumors from one laboratory mouse to another: If it can happen in mice, why not humans? Actually, the mice used in those experiments are either specially inbred to be genetically identical, or they have had treatments to make their immune systems powerless.

There are two sexually transmitted viruses that have been linked to cancer: the human immunodeficiency virus (HIV), which causes AIDS, and the human papilloma virus (HPV), which causes genital warts. A person who contracted HIV or HPV during sex may indeed increase his or her risk of developing a few types of cancer. For people with HIV, there has been an increased risk of cancers such as Kaposi's sarcoma, non-Hodgkin's lymphoma, testicular cancer, and squamous cell cancers of the anus or cervix. HPV is suspected to cause cancer of the cervix and vulva in women and perhaps, once in a while, to play a role in cancer of the penis.

Cancer and Divorce

Probably every person who reads this book has heard stories about cancer patients whose spouses abandoned them or has personally seen or experienced such a situation. A variety of surveys, however, have not found any unusual divorce rates after one spouse has cancer. In fact, the majority of couples rate the cancer as bringing them closer together. These findings hold true even when the patients surveyed developed sexual problems related to cancer treatment. Cancer can be a reminder not to take health or loved ones for granted.

Remember that about half of all marriages in the United States end in divorce. When someone leaves a spouse who has cancer, it stands out like a mental headline, leading people to overestimate the role of cancer in breaking up marriages. In my years of counseling cancer patients, I have found I can often predict which relationships are likely to break up. They are couples who already had trouble communicating and resolving conflicts before cancer was ever diagnosed. Going through cancer treatment, with its financial and emotional stresses, becomes the final straw. Although the stereotype is that the healthy partner leaves the one who is ill, sometimes it is the patient who gets fed up with the lack of support received during the illness and says, "That's it. Now I've had enough."

Cancer and Feeling Attractive

Having cancer not only can change people's actual physical appearance, it also can alter how attractive they feel and how others look at them. In the past, cancer was often regarded as an unclean disease, and people with cancer were shunned, much like the discrimination today against people with HIV. Even well-informed people still sometimes overreact to cancer.

> Sally had just had a baby when her husband, Tim, was diagnosed with Hodgkin's disease. She was very supportive of him during his chemotherapy, but Tim confided to one of his young nurses that things were not so good at home. He said that Sally no longer was willing to have sex with him. With Tim's permission, his social worker spoke to Sally, who admitted that her desire for Tim had disappeared. "I feel really guilty, but I just don't feel like having sex with him right now. Without his hair, and with all the weight he's lost, he just doesn't seem like the Tim I married."

Of course, some types of cancer treatment leave visible and permanent changes. Body changes that are not seen by the casual observer but are obvious to a lover include those that result from a mastectomy, losing a testicle, or having a urinary ostomy or colostomy.

The most devastating physical changes are usually those that can be seen by everyone—facial scars, an amputated arm or leg, spinal damage necessitating the use of a wheelchair, or a laryngectomy. Public changes in body image do not leave you a choice about confronting your illness with strangers or casual acquaintances. Unfortunately, having a visible disability also leaves men and women vulnerable to discrimination or abuse from ignorant people who may stare, ask rude questions, or make ugly remarks. Even people who have healthy self-esteem may need extra support to cope with such experiences (see "Let's Face It" in Resources under Information Networks, Cancer, Specific Types).

In my work with couples over the years, I have been impressed by the supportiveness most partners show where body image is concerned. Typically a man or woman who undergoes cancer surgery is far more upset and frightened than the partner about the impact of physical scars on sexual attraction.

If you have or had cancer and fear a partner would no longer find you attractive, try this exercise to see the situation from a partner's perspective—Find a few private moments and close your eyes. Imagine that you never had cancer, but that your partner is instead the one with the illness. Picture your partner with a body change parallel to the one that bothers you. (If you do not have a sexual partner right now, think of someone you were close to in the past.) Imagine making love to your partner with this physical change. Would you be turned off? Could you still enjoy sex in spite of your partner's cancer? Would you stop having sex or end the relationship?

Typically, we judge ourselves more harshly than others do.

Depression and Your Sexual Feelings

Most people who go through cancer treatment have periods of feeling depressed. These periods are usually temporary and lessen over time. A smaller group of people experience a major clinical depression—a mood disorder marked not only by feeling depressed, but also by loss of pleasure in life, difficulty sleeping, changes in appetite for food, feeling lethargic or unusually restless, having trouble concentrating and remembering things, feeling guilty and worthless, and having many thoughts about suicide or death. Loss of interest in sex and decreased satisfaction with sex are also common in depression. Symptoms of depression are considered significant if they last for more than two weeks.

Sometimes it is difficult to separate these symptoms from the side effects of cancer and its treatments. For example, people on chemotherapy often have changes in their appetite for food and either lose or gain weight. During cancer treatment, people may feel tired or have trouble concentrating. Thoughts about death or dying can be evoked by fears of cancer progressing. Deciding if someone is depressed or just having a normal reaction to cancer treatment can be difficult. However, true depression is probably present if the person shows a severe and lasting change in mood, in ability to enjoy life, and in mental alertness. Depression becomes more common when cancer advances and normal daily activities are limited.

Sometimes a man or woman complains of loss of interest in sex when the underlying problem is really depression. Because society views depression as a weakness, it may be more socially acceptable to focus on a change in sexual desire.

Don was only 38 and the father of three children when a nasty cough led to a chest X ray and diagnosis of incurable lung cancer. As Don began to grow weaker, he refused to talk about dying and spent his days lying in bed and watching TV. His biggest complaint was that he could not have good erections anymore, so he asked to see a urologist. The urologist gave Don a vacuum constriction device (see Chapter 11), a small pump that would help him get better erections before having intercourse. Don complained, however, that using the pump made him feel like a robot instead of a man. Only after Don's wife talked in detail to the medical team about his behavior did they realize that he was actually quite depressed. Don's mood improved when the home hospice team became involved in his care. They prescribed an antidepressant for him and provided counseling. Don did use his vacuum device to stay sexually active until he became too ill.

In Sickness and in Health: Switching between Caretaker and Lover

One common pattern that emerges during cancer treatment is that a healthy partner becomes the caretaker of the ill one. Sometimes the ill partner needs help with the most private of functions, such as toileting, care of a surgical incision, emptying vomit trays, or bathing. It is difficult then to switch gears and feel like lovers again.

When a person reacts to the cancer by acting helpless and childlike, caretaker patterns can get entrenched. Instead of learning how to care for his own urinary ostomy, a man expects his wife to do it. A woman stays in bed all day, calling family members to bring her a soft drink or a magazine to read. After a while, sympathy turns to frustration, and the healthy partner alternately feels guilty and dreams of a solo trip to the Bahamas. Either way, sexual desire for the cancer victim is not on the menu. Men or women who let cancer turn them into invalids may have always had a tendency to react to stress by giving up. Illness tends to exaggerate typical personality styles.

Men, Women, and Cancer

Men and women are brought up to deal with crises in different ways. Men are taught to keep their emotions under control and take action to fix things. An advantage of this approach is that problems get solved. A disadvantage is that the family may see a man as withdrawn or rejecting because he is trying to hide his fear and hopelessness.

When cancer interferes with sexual function, men often express fears that they will no longer be fully male. A loss of sexual abilities is often coupled with damage to earning power—two aspects of manhood that are key in the United States. Despite the anguish men may feel, their belief that seeking help is weak often keeps them from getting treatment for problems with sexuality or infertility.

Women have more permission to express feelings and are mandated to provide tender loving care to others. On the positive side, women's ability to cry or to talk out fears is very helpful in coping with cancer. On the negative side, women often have trouble taking care of themselves when they are the patients because they are so used to putting other family members first.

Women also talk about a loss of femininity after mastectomy or hysterectomy, for example. Many of women's sexual concerns, however, center around fear of losing a relationship, either because of loss of physical beauty or because of inability to satisfy a partner sexually.

Because men and women generally have such different strategies for coping, partners sometimes have trouble providing support for each other during cancer treatment. A woman who is ill wants validation for her emotional pain—someone to say he understands how she feels and to hold her lovingly. Instead, she often gets a husband who tells her, "Cheer up! It will all turn out okay." A man who has cancer often wants a woman who will distract him by joking or by planning enjoyable activities. He may be dismayed by a wife who wants to talk tearfully about her fears of losing him.

Infertility after Cancer and Your Sexuality

As frightening and disruptive as cancer is, an extra emotional burden is added when cancer treatment interferes with plans to have children. Grief over loss of fertility can also spill over into a man's or woman's sex life, even when cancer treatment has not damaged sexual function directly.

Mona had just married for the first time at age 35 when her leukemia was diagnosed. She and her husband had thrown away their contraceptives on the wedding night, ready to start trying immediately for a pregnancy. Instead, they were faced with the prospect of a bone marrow transplant. Mona's oncologist warned her that the high-dose chemotherapy that would be used to kill off her own bone marrow was almost 100 percent likely to produce a permanent menopause. She would be able to take estrogen after her recovery to prevent hot flashes and vaginal dryness, but there was no way to protect her eggs from the destructive impact of the chemotherapy drugs.

Even though Mona felt lucky that her bone marrow transplant was success-ful, it was very difficult for her to enjoy sex even a year or two afterward. Every time she and her husband made love, Mona felt empty and sad because she knew pregnancy was impossible. She could not separate the idea of sexual pleasure from her wish for a child.

Thoughts and feelings related to cancer often interfere with enjoying sex. Yet, confronting cancer is also a reminder to enjoy each day and not take life for granted. The rest of this section focuses on how you can enjoy your sex life again after cancer.

2

Am I Normal? Men's
Sexual Health

In order to understand how cancer treatment can interfere with a man's sex life, it is necessary to understand the basics of normal sexuality. Although the facts of life for men appear simple—get an erection, keep it, and ejaculate—the actual male response is quite complex. Not only the brain, but several parts of the nervous system control each of the crucial phases of men's sexual function: desire, arousal, orgasm, and resolution. Men themselves often wonder "Am I normal?" even if they are in good health. Men tend to compare themselves to their peers, often overestimating the other guy's sexual success. Here are some of the most common questions I hear from men, along with the answers:

Question: How long is the average man's penis?
Answer: About 5 to 6 inches.
Question: How long does the penetration part of intercourse last for the average man?
Answer: About 7 to 10 minutes.
Question: How often does the average man have sex?
Answer: In men age 18 to 50, roughly a third of men have sex less than monthly, a third have sex a few times a month, and a third have sex twice a week or more. On the average, men over 50 have sex less often than younger men.
Question: How many men have erection problems?
Answer: For men under 40, about 10 percent of men have erection problems. With age, problems become more common, affecting 50 percent of men by age 70.

When I started out as a psychologist working in a cancer center, I dis-

covered by interviewing men who survived cancer that their sexual problems were very specific. For example, doctors and patients often assumed
that without an erection, no sexual pleasure would be possible. Yet many
men who could not get firm erections after cancer treatment still had
excellent sensation on the penis and, with the right kind of stimulation,
could reach orgasm. Other men had the sensation of orgasm but did not
ejaculate any semen. Some men had little desire for sex, but if they made
a real effort to get in the mood, they could achieve erections and reach
orgasm.

To understand how cancer treatment can cause sexual problems, it is
necessary to have a working knowledge of a man's normal sexual function
and the changes that are typical with aging.

Sexual Desire: What Is This Thing Called Lust?

Sexual desire is usually the first event in a man's sexual response, and also
the aspect that is hardest to define. Sexual desire is being in the mood for
sex, feeling horny (although not necessarily having an erection), or being
frustrated by a lack of sex.

Although there is no physical way to measure desire, sexual feelings are
linked to testosterone, often called the male sex hormone. At puberty,
special cells in each testicle, called Leydig cells, begin producing more
testosterone. In response, a boy's voice deepens, his penis grows to full
size, and his body hair and beard develop. During a man's whole adult life,
testosterone circulates in his bloodstream and acts in his brain to help
him feel a desire for sex. Testosterone also may play a role in skin sensitivity to sexual caressing on the penis. A man only needs a minimum
amount of testosterone to have a normal sex life. Despite many articles
and TV shows suggesting that taking extra testosterone will enhance a
man's desire, excess testosterone does little or nothing for sexual pleasure
or performance, even in older men.

Other chemicals in the brain, called neurotransmitters, also influence
sexual desire. They carry messages from one nerve cell to another. Which
neurotransmitters are crucial to sexual desire or the exact areas of the brain
involved are not really known. It is known that the ability to feel interest
in sex does not depend just on chemistry, but also on a man's life experience.

Stan was only 52 when trouble with urination led him to seek medical advice.
He was found to have prostate cancer that had already spread to his lymph

nodes. As a treatment, he took monthly hormone shots that stopped his testicles from making testosterone. Stan's doctor told him to expect to lose interest in sex as a side effect of treatment. Over several months, however, Stan was surprised and relieved to find that his desire did not completely disappear. Although it took more time and stimulation to get an erection, watching an X-rated video or talking about sexual fantasies with his wife helped. Stan's wife was also comfortable spending a few minutes on hand caressing or giving him oral sex. Because of his hormone treatment, it took him longer than before to reach orgasm, and he only produced a few drops of semen. If you think of testosterone as the "grease on the wheel" of desire, Stan's strong sex drive and excellent marriage kept him trucking.

Sexual Arousal: The Excitement Mounts

With sexual excitement, blood flow increases to the penis and the rest of the genitals. As a result, the penis becomes firm and erect. Physical arousal is usually matched by a sense of mental excitement and strong sensations of erotic pleasure from caressing of the body's sensitive areas. The cross section of a man's pelvis in Figure 2.1 shows the structure of the penis, prostate, testicles, and other reproductive organs.

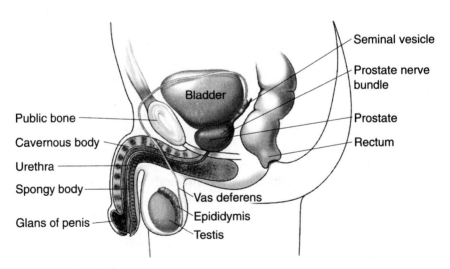

Figure 2.1   Cross section of the male pelvis

The Penis

You may be happy to know that the penis is actually twice as long as you thought! The part of the penis that hangs down from the body is just the outer half. The chambers of the penis extend backward into the body, over the area where the scrotal sac and testicles lie. The penis has three inner chambers. Two run lengthwise, side by side, to form the top of the shaft. Called cavernous bodies, they are filled with soft, spongy tissue that includes muscle cells, spaces, and many tiny blood vessels. Each cavernous body has a small artery to supply it with blood. The cavernous bodies are surrounded by several layers of tough tissue that are crucial in the erection process.

Along the bottom of the shaft runs the spongy body, a separate chamber centered around the urethra—a tube that begins at the urinary bladder, travels through the prostate, and ends at the tip of the penis. The urethra carries both urine and semen out of the body. The spongy body also contains spongy tissue, which fans out at the tip of the penis to form the glans, or head of the penis.

Erection

Erection takes place in a series of steps. While the penis is soft, the muscle cells inside remain tensed so that blood cannot enter the spaces in the cavernous bodies (picture a dry sponge). When the nervous system signals an erection to begin, the muscular tissue relaxes, and the arteries send more blood into the cavernous bodies. The penis swells as blood fills up its spaces, like a sponge filling with water. The tough layers of tissue surrounding the spongy areas limit the swelling, so that as more blood flows in, pressure builds and the penis becomes stiff. As the penis swells, this tough casing squeezes against a series of veins, sealing them off to prevent blood from draining out of the cavernous bodies. Extra blood also fills the head of the penis, which enlarges, becomes a deeper color, and warms to the touch.

The Erection Nerve Center

The nerves that direct blood to flow into the penis are the final link in a pathway that begins in the brain and continues down the spinal cord, with nerves exiting into the pelvis around the level of the lower back. These nerves, part of the involuntary, or sympathetic and parasympathetic, nervous system, run between the back of the prostate and the rectum (see Figure 2.1). They continue along the urethra and enter the penis. The nerves around the prostate are easy to damage during pelvic cancer treatment. (This will be discussed in Chapter 10.)

The Male Orgasm: Not an Anticlimax

If sexual stimulation continues, a man will usually reach orgasm—a sensation of extreme pleasure. Orgasm has several different ingredients: pleasure, emission, and ejaculation.

The *pleasure* comes with a burst of activity in the brain. Orgasm is triggered in the brain via signals from the sensory nerves that sense touch on the skin of the genital area.

Although semen spurting out might add to a man's pleasure, it is a separate event with two stages of its own. The first is *emission*, which men describe as the "feeling of no return"—the sensation that an orgasm is about to happen. During emission, the semen cocktail is being mixed. Most of the milky fluid that makes up semen is produced by the seminal vesicles (see Figure 2.1), two small sacs located behind the prostate. The rest of the fluid comes from the prostate itself. The smooth muscle of the prostate and seminal vesicles squeezes together, mixing the seminal fluid. Ripe sperm cells are added in from the epididymis, the area where they are stored. The fluid oozes into the top of the urethra, ready for the moment of ejaculation. At the same time, a valve between the bladder and prostate shuts tightly so that the fluid must squirt forward when ejaculation begins. Emission is controlled by a part of the nervous system called the sympathetic nerves. These nerves are not the same as those that carry messages from the skin.

The sensory nerves *do* control the second part of orgasm, however, *ejaculation*. During ejaculation, muscles at the base of the penis squeeze rhythmically, forcing the semen to spurt out of the urethra. Some types of cancer treatment leave men with a dry orgasm that feels normal but has no release of semen (see Chapter 12).

Resolution: Nature's Rest Period

After sexual arousal, whether or not an orgasm occurs, resolution takes place. The nerves and blood vessels involved in erection return to their normal, unexcited state. During arousal, blood flows into the skin of the scrotal sac, creating a feeling of fullness. After orgasm, blood is quickly diverted back out of the penis and genital area. If a man gets aroused but does not reach orgasm, he may feel a crampy sensation in his scrotum because the blood vessels remain full for up to an hour or two before blood circulation normalizes. Although men complain about this discomfort to make women feel guilty, it is no more harmful than a headache!

Men have a *refractory phase* after orgasm—a resting period that the body demands. During this time, a man may have difficulty getting another erection and, even if he is able to get excited, will not be able to reach orgasm. The refractory phase lengthens with age. A 17-year-old may be able to ejaculate and continue sexual activity with barely a pause to catch his breath. A 77-year-old may need a couple of days to recover from one orgasm enough to have another. Young men who ejaculate quickly may have sex twice in quick succession to satisfy their partners. As men get older and have a longer refractory phase (and, thus, less frequent sex), they typically need to focus on having a quality experience each time they begin sex.

Although the physical basis of the refractory phase is not well understood, chemicals produced in the brain are responsible for it. As you can imagine, pharmaceutical companies would love to invent a drug to shorten the refractory phase, but so far they have had no luck.

Sex and Aging in Men: It's Not All Downhill

Men's sexual responses do change with age. Teenagers get erections automatically (in fact, often when it is embarrassing and irrelevant, like in the middle of math class). For 40-, 50-, and 60-year-olds, it takes longer to develop a full erection, and direct touch to the skin of the penis may be required. Getting older gives men a great rationale to ask partners to take the lead or to provide more caressing of the penis during lovemaking.

Another advantage of aging is that it gives men greater ability to hold off ejaculation. Lasting longer can add to both partners' satisfaction and pleasure.

When men of different ages are surveyed, there appears a trend showing that older men feel less desire for sex and have sex less often. Much of this decline may be related to health problems that interfere with sex or to losing a partner through death or divorce. Erection problems become more common, affecting about half of men by age 70. Men who are diabetic, who have high blood pressure or heart disease, or who take medications for these and other conditions are more likely to develop erection problems. Aging and the diseases that go with it affect the muscle cells and blood vessels in the penis. The tissue may not relax easily to let blood flow in, or too much blood can drain out during erection. Sometimes the delicate nerves involved in erection are also damaged.

Nevertheless, there is no true male menopause. Most men stay sexually active all their lives and have all the testosterone they need, even in old age.

Now that we have looked at male sexuality, we are ready to review the facts of life for women.

3

Greater Expectations: Women's Sexual Health

The most striking thing about women's sexual health in the United States in the past century is the change regarding expectations for female sexual pleasure. Attitudes have certainly shifted from pre–World War I primness to today's ceaseless media messages to women to get the most out of sex. Women's actual behavior has also changed, with more women having sex outside of marriage and starting their sex lives at younger ages. One of the best predictors of a woman's capacity for sexual pleasure is the decade of her birth—the more recently she was born, the more likely she is to be orgasmic.

Men's and women's bodies respond to sexual stimulation in many parallel ways. The hormone testosterone stimulates sexual desire in both sexes. Just as blood flow to the penis produces an erection, increased blood flow to the vaginal walls with arousal enlarges and lubricates the vagina. The clitoris is shaped like a tiny penis and has a similar sensitivity to erotic touch. During orgasm, genital muscles contract in the same exact rhythm in men and women.

Yet men's and women's sexual response is also different, in ways probably determined as much by society as by biology. Men's sexual satisfaction is closely tied to having firm erections and frequent sexual intercourse. Women's sexual satisfaction is more strongly related to relationship happiness.

Women often go on having sex for their partner's sake, even if cancer treatment interferes with sexual desire and pleasure. Older women in particular, however, rarely seek help for a sexual problem unless it prevents their satisfying a partner.

When Mae was growing up in rural Alabama, the church was the center of her African-American family's life. There was no drinking, dancing, or swearing, and certainly no talk at home about sex. Mae knew something about sex from growing up on a farm, but when she married Joe at age 20, the reality of erections and intercourse were pretty shocking at first. Mae never got a lot of enjoyment from foreplay, since she never felt right about having her breasts or genital area stroked. Joe typically only could make intercourse last for a couple of minutes. But sex was important to Mae, even at 66, when her uterine cancer was diagnosed. When intercourse became painful, she asked her surgeon for help, even though she found it very humiliating and embarrassing to discuss her personal business with a man young enough to be her son. "Don't mistake me," she told him. "I could live fine without sex for the rest of my life. But it isn't fair to my husband."

Cancer treatment also might bring an early menopause to young women or affect older women's decisions about taking hormones to ease the symptoms of natural menopause. These issues have no male parallel. First, I'll review facts about the normal sexual response in women, and then discuss the impact of menopause on sexuality.

Women's Desire: Hormones and Fantasy

Sexual desire for women depends on emotional factors such as a yen for a particular partner, comfort with sexual fantasy, and feeling attractive. As in men, testosterone and related hormones (called androgens) act in women's brains to promote sexual desire. About half of the androgens circulating in a woman's bloodstream are made by her ovaries. The other half are produced in the adrenal glands. (One adrenal gland is located over each kidney.) Estrogen and progesterone, the other two hormones made in the ovaries, regulate a woman's menstrual cycle, but have little influence on her interest in sex.

Women's androgen levels are much lower than men's. Only a tiny amount of testosterone is needed to maintain good sexual desire, but the exact lower limit of "normal" is not really known.

Female Excitement: A Hidden Flowering

When women become sexually aroused, blood rushes into the genital area. Many women have never looked at their genital area in a mirror and have only a vague idea of their "equipment." Figure 3.1 shows the outside of the **vulva**. Each woman has the same parts, although women's vulvas vary quite a bit in skin color and shape (see *Femalia* in Resources under Books). The outer lips *(labia majora)* are filled with spongy tissue and act as a cushion to protect the delicate and sensitive inner lips *(labia minora)*. Some women's inner lips are small and regular, but others have longer lips that form small ruffles of tissue. The size and appearance of the inner lips often change after a woman gives birth.

Where the inner lips meet at the bottom, a small slit marks the vaginal opening. At the upper junction of the inner lips, a small hood of skin is found. Underneath the hood is a round bump, the head of the clitoris. The clitoris is actually shaped like a tiny penis and has a shaft hidden underneath its hood. The hood itself is the female version of a foreskin (the loose skin over the head of the penis in men who are not circumcised). The head of the clitoris is so well supplied with nerve endings that many women find direct caressing too intense and prefer to be touched over the clitoral hood. The opening of the urethra (the tube from the urinary bladder to the outside) can be found between the clitoris and the vaginal entrance. The urethra, vagina, and anal canal are three separate passageways.

When a woman begins to get sexually aroused, the skin of her vulva turns a deeper pink or red color, and the clitoris swells slightly. With more

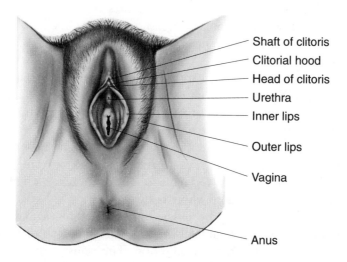

Figure 3.1   The vulva

stimulation, the clitoris actually pulls in closer to the body, so that the small ridge of its shaft is more difficult to feel under the hood. The most important changes with excitement occur inside the vagina, however, where they cannot be seen. The thick muscular walls of the vagina fill with blood. The vagina becomes a third deeper than in its unexcited state. The deepest area balloons out, while the vaginal walls closest to the entrance become plump and firm. The special lining of the vagina produces clear droplets of slippery fluid, similar to beads of sweat.

All of these changes prepare the vagina for intercourse. The vagina is moist and open, making penetration easier. The outer part of the vagina can hug the penis, creating pleasurable friction on the most sensitive areas of the vaginal walls (although the clitoris is twice as sensitive as the inside of the vagina). The deep part of the vagina expands so that the thrusting penis does not hammer against tender organs inside the pelvis.

The Female Orgasm

Why do many women have trouble reaching orgasm? Why do women have orgasms at all? Some researchers believe that women's orgasms were built in during human evolution. After all, a woman who enjoys sex is more likely to get pregnant and pass down her genes. Others say there is no rhyme or reason for female orgasms. They just happen to occur because of the parallels between men's and women's bodies. Some speculate that the muscle contractions of a woman's orgasm suck sperm cells through the cervix and into her uterus to meet a ripe egg, but this theory has never been proved.

Authorities on sex have also argued about what type of orgasm is normal for women. Some claim that orgasms during intercourse are unique and more natural, pleasurable, mature, or complete than orgasms from other types of sexual stimulation. The one thing we know is that for a majority of women, orgasms from penile thrusting in the vagina occur less easily and rapidly than orgasms from caressing the clitoris. Many women say that orgasms from clitoral caressing feel more focused and intense, whereas those during intercourse are a more whole body experience.

During a woman's orgasm, the muscles surrounding the vaginal entrance and anal area contract rhythmically and messages of pleasure are sent to the brain by nerves that register sensation. The walls of the uterus also squeeze rhythmically, although most women are not aware of extra sensations in the uterus. Uterine contractions are controlled by the involuntary nervous system. The vaginal and anal contractions during orgasm and the feeling of pleasure are controlled by sensory nerves. It is unclear whether women have a two-phase orgasm similar to men's (see Chapter 2), although subjectively, most women can identify a feeling of "no return" before their orgasm begins.

Women do not ejaculate a fluid or produce extra vaginal lubrication at the moment of orgasm. In 1982, the book *The G-Spot and Other Recent Discoveries about Human Sexuality* suggested that some women do produce a spurt of clear fluid at orgasm from the urethra. Most scientists now believe that this liquid is actually urine. Women whose pelvic muscles and ligaments have been stretched by childbirth or damaged by surgery often develop mild stress incontinence—losing a small amount of urine if they cough, jump, and so on. These women may also urinate a small amount during orgasm. Urine is a sterile fluid and is not harmful or dirty. If a woman is worried about losing urine during orgasm, she can often prevent it by emptying her bladder just before starting lovemaking.

Unlike men, women have no refractory phase after orgasm. It is physically possible for a woman to have a whole series of orgasms, separated by a few seconds or several minutes. Although multiple orgasms have been held out as a sexual goal by books and magazines, they are not necessarily superior to one orgasm. Women vary in what they enjoy. Many women say that one intense orgasm is enough and that they do not feel like having another right away. Often, women enjoy sex even if no orgasm occurs.

Resolution: Time for Afterplay

After an orgasm, blood flow reverts quickly to its normal pattern. The vaginal walls collapse onto each other and the vaginal lining stops producing lubrication. When a woman gets aroused but does not reach orgasm, she might notice a crampy or full feeling in her pelvic area. This is often called *pelvic congestion* and is similar to the aching men often report around their scrotum after prolonged sexual excitement. Women often focus on resolution as a time to enjoy the cuddling and intimacy of afterplay.

Menopause: What Is It?

At menopause, a woman's menstrual periods stop because her ovaries no longer produce the hormones estrogen and progesterone. A woman might have her uterus removed surgically and, thus, have no menstrual bleeding; but as long as she has at least one working ovary, she is not truly in menopause. The most typical symptom of menopause is hot flashes—a sensation of heat and flushing, often including sweating. Hot flashes tend to happen most often at night. If they disturb a woman's sleep, she might feel irritable and tired.

Contrary to the stereotype that women become depressed and highly emotional at menopause, large studies of healthy women in the community show that most women have a positive experience and are relieved to be free of menstruation. Hot flashes and other symptoms of menopause are only mildly annoying. Women who do become depressed at midlife are often under unusual stress. Worries about a mate or children are their most common concerns.

The average age of menopause is 51, but reaching menopause anywhere in the late forties to early fifties is considered normal. If a woman is not sure that she is in menopause, blood tests for the hormones FSH (follicle stimulating hormone) or estradiol (a strong form of estrogen) can reveal her status.

Menopause and Sex

The most common sexual problem related to menopause is vaginal dryness. Because of the loss of estrogen, the vaginal walls lose some of their blood supply, becoming less stretchy and plump. The vaginal lining becomes thin and fragile, producing less lubrication with sexual arousal. If these changes are severe, a woman might find that her vagina feels tight and dry, even when she feels highly excited. Thrusting in the vagina might burn. After intercourse, she might notice either light spotting of blood from small tears in the vaginal lining or vaginal irritation that can last for a day or two.

Infections of the vagina and urinary tract also are common sources of discomfort during sex after menopause. The vagina has a less acid pH, making conditions right for monilial yeast infections. With thinning tissue around the vulva, the urethra gets more easily irritated during sexual activity. Bacteria that find their way into the urethra and bladder then are more likely to grow and cause a urinary tract infection. For women who use replacement estrogens, the vaginal changes of menopause quickly can be reversed, however. Women who do not use estrogen can often benefit from water-based vaginal lubricants (see Chapter 14).

After menopause, the ovaries continue producing androgens, but the amount trickles off over the years. The adrenal glands maintain the same output as before. Despite the falling amount of androgens circulating in the blood, desire problems are the exception rather than the rule after natural menopause.

When women lose both ovaries suddenly, however, for example as part of cancer treatment, lack of androgens might sometimes trigger sexual problems (see Chapter 8). When menopause occurs prematurely, all its symptoms tend to be more severe. Women may have more hot flashes, more severe vaginal changes, and more mood changes.

Menopause, Estrogen Replacement, and Women's Health

Women who have had cancer often want to live as healthy and natural a life as possible. Such lifestyle choices as following a diet low in fat and high in fiber, getting regular exercise, not smoking, and not using alcohol to excess can benefit every woman. To women who are menopausal after cancer, whether the change of life was brought on by treatment or just because of the natural aging process, the idea of taking estrogen sounds risky and might seem artificial, or against nature's plan. But women were probably not designed to live to an average age of 80, including 30 years of menopause, and living without estrogen brings health risks. The loss of estrogen increases a woman's risk of two important health problems: osteoporosis and cardiovascular disease.

Osteoporosis is a condition defined by thinning of the bones. In all women, bones gradually lose calcium and become more fragile with age. Women who are small-boned and fair-skinned and who have smoked, have been heavy drinkers, or have a family history of osteoporosis are at higher risk for problems. Osteoporosis is a major cause of death in elderly women because of the complications (such as pneumonia) that often develop after a broken hip. Osteoporosis also contributes to back pain from thinned or fractured vertebrae in the spine. Women with osteoporosis often lose some height or develop "widow's hump" (a curvature of the upper spine).

Although a diet rich in calcium and getting regular, weight-bearing exercise help women maintain bone strength, these strategies are not nearly as effective after menopause as estrogen replacement in preventing osteoporosis. Newer, nonhormonal medications to prevent osteoporosis are also available. (For more information, contact The National Osteoporosis Foundation—see Resources under Information Networks.)

Cardiovascular disease remains the most common cause of death in women. Although men are more likely to have heart attacks before age 50, rates of heart disease in women rise quickly after menopause. Estrogen protects against heart disease. It increases the levels of high density, or "good," cholesterol and also enhances blood flow to vital organs, including the heart. Women who take replacement estrogen after menopause have fewer heart attacks than those not on hormones.

Replacement estrogen is very effective at low doses in keeping bones strong, protecting the heart, reversing menopausal damage to the vagina, and stopping hot flashes. Estrogen can be taken in the form of a pill, a patch that is worn on the abdomen for several days at a time, or in a vaginal cream. Some women feel safer using a vaginal cream because they see it as a local treatment for vaginal dryness and irritation. The vagina is richly supplied with blood vessels, however, and the hormones from the cream do enter the general bloodstream, sometimes providing a larger dose of estrogen than a pill would.

Several large, long-term studies of healthy women have showed that those who take replacement estrogen live longer because they suffer less osteoporosis and heart disease. Women who take estrogen for several years do have an increased risk of cancer of the uterus. Women who still have their uterus are usually advised to combine replacement estrogen with some form of progesterone. Progesterone pills are the most commonly prescribed. Progesterone counteracts the tendency of estrogen to promote overgrowth of the uterine lining. The type of uterine cancer usually seen in women who take estrogen is slow-growing and easy to find early with a yearly gynecological examination. It often causes vaginal bleeding, which should prompt a woman to seek medical advice right away. Although uterine cancer related to replacement estrogen must be treated with a hysterectomy, it rarely is a cause of death in older women.

Recent studies suggest a small increase in the risk of breast cancer for women who take replacement estrogen after menopause. Adding progesterone does not help reduce the impact of estrogen on breast tissue. The breast cancer risk is small, however, compared to the benefits of estrogen replacement in prolonging women's lives. Estrogen might even have a protective effect against colon cancer.

Young women who become prematurely menopausal after treatment for cancer of the cervix, leukemia, or Hodgkin's disease should strongly consider taking estrogen to keep their bones strong and protect their cardiovascular systems. Each woman should discuss her personal risks for cancer, osteoporosis, and heart disease with her physician in making a decision whether to take estrogen after menopause. Women who have already had breast cancer are typically advised never to take estrogen, but thoughts about this are changing (see Chapter 23 for a discussion of the pros and cons).

It is important not only to understand what is normal sexually for women and men, but also to be able to talk about sexual desires and problems with your partner. The next two chapters suggest ways to communicate about sex and then take action to make your sex life better when cancer has interfered.

4

Getting the Words Out: Talking about Sex

Being able to talk about sex with your partner is a crucial step in recovering a satisfying sex life after cancer treatment. If your sex life has been interrupted or you have developed problems experiencing sexual desire and pleasure, you might need to try a variety of strategies to overcome the barriers built during your illness. Some remedies only involve changing your internal images or exploring your own sensations in private. Most techniques, however, require some teamwork with your partner. Thus, getting back to normal might mean talking more frankly about sex than you ever have in the past.

Patients often tell me, "I want sex to be spontaneous." They mean that the desire for sex should hit both partners simultaneously like a bolt from the blue. Initiation should be wordless and mutual, with instant understanding between mates about what will take place. It certainly should not be necessary to negotiate about safer sex or to guide each other during lovemaking. Although telepathic passion is not a realistic expectation, many men and women feel that talking during sex breaks the mood and is unnecessary.

Perhaps you have always had an easy time discussing your sexual likes and dislikes. If so, you are ahead of the game. Most men and women have trouble talking about their sexual feelings. Have you ever told a sexual partner exactly how you like to be touched genitally, what you think about during lovemaking, or, even more taboo, if and how you masturbate?

Having cancer might bring up new issues that leave you tongue-tied. Do you still excite your partner when chemotherapy has made you hairless? If your erections are no longer firm, would your partner be willing to have orgasms through hand or oral caressing instead of during intercourse?

30

have orgasms through hand or oral caressing instead of during intercourse? What is the best way to use a vaginal lubricant so that it does not interrupt the mood of your lovemaking? Do you want your partner to caress your reconstructed breast? How can you keep your ostomy appliance out of the way during sex? Should you use a condom during oral sex to avoid exposing your partner to chemotherapy drugs in your semen?

This chapter will give you suggestions on how to say things that seem unspeakable. First, however, consider the state of sexual communication in your current sex life. Over my years as a sex therapist, I have found that couples fall into some typical categories when it comes to discussing sexual matters. I have labeled these categories:

- Name, Rank, and Serial Number
- Mount Vesuvius
- The Average Guys
- Sexual Athletes

Name, Rank, and Serial Number

This communication style can be summed up in two words—no communication. In my experience, many couples in this group grew up in the first half of the century when sex was still taboo, although younger couples also can be tongue-tied about sex. Often neither partner has had much experience with lovemaking. They learn about each other's bodies through trial and error—and all too often the errors make sex into a lifelong trial.

> Bud and Joyce had been married for forty-three years when his colon cancer was diagnosed. After undergoing surgery and radiation therapy, Bud was left with a colostomy and an erection problem. He and Joyce discontinued their sex life and probably never would have mentioned the fact if a young resident assigned to their case had not brought it up. Bud's reply was, "Oh, that part of our lives is over now."
>
> When the doctor pressed on, Bud and Joyce disclosed that they had been sexually active perhaps twice a month until the cancer was diagnosed. Bud had always initiated sex, and foreplay had never lasted more than a couple of minutes. Joyce was taking estrogen replacement but said she had used a lubricant to make sex comfortable because the amount of touching and kissing she got from her husband was just not enough to arouse her for intercourse. Her response surprised Bud. "I always felt like you just wanted to get things over with," he said.
>
> Joyce said she was brought up to believe that her husband would know how

to please her in bed. She never felt it was right to criticize Bud, even though his touch was always too rough. Not surprisingly, Joyce had never experienced an orgasm, except once in a while when she had a dream about sex and woke up right at the moment of her climax. She had never looked at her genital area in the mirror, and neither she nor Bud was sure where to find the clitoris.

Couples with little sexual communication often develop a routine in their lovemaking. The same types of caressing take place in their typical order. If any orgasms occur, they happen during penis-in-vagina intercourse. Couples like Joyce and Bud rarely experiment with hand or oral caressing to orgasm as a way to enjoy lovemaking if a cancer-related sexual problem makes intercourse difficult. There is little variety or flexibility in their sexual activities. If traditional sex will not work, they give up.

Mount Vesuvius

This type of couple has always had a problem with sex. They might not discuss it often, but when they do the explosion of anger and blaming is as predictable as a volcanic eruption. If cancer treatment interferes with sex, it just helps the pressure to build.

Nora's cancer of the cervix was successfully treated with a radical hysterectomy. Most women are able to return to a normal sex life with good sensation and ability to reach orgasm after this surgery, despite the loss of some vaginal depth. Nora complained, however, that she "felt nothing" when she tried to have sex. She was referred for sexual counseling, accompanied by her husband, Eddie.

Eddie was an imposing man, now running to flab. Nora was petite but looked older than her age. "If I knew what this operation was going to do to me as a woman," she began, "I think I would rather have died." Eddie rolled his eyes and snorted.

Nora raised her voice. "You see what I put up with? If it weren't for him, I wouldn't be here at all today! I wouldn't have cancer to begin with if he hadn't given me warts all over my private parts—filthy warts that he got from the whores he plays around with!" Eddie looked as though he were going to protest. He shook his head wearily, but Nora continued, "He knows! I was a nineteen-year-old virgin when I married him."

"Yeah, and you made up for it double in the last eighteen years," Eddie interjected.

"Like hell, I did. I haven't touched another man besides you, except when I finally couldn't stand it and left for a year."

"Yeah, and how many did you have then?" Eddie seized his opportunity.

"Doctor!" Nora interrupted him. "I'm here because my husband tells me that, since my operation, sex with me gives him no pleasure at all." The psychologist tried to clarify whether the loss of pleasure was on Eddie's side or Nora's. Nora explained that she got about as much pleasure from intercourse as she always had, that is to say, not much, because Eddie knows nothing about how to please a woman and ejaculates almost as soon as he enters her. It was Eddie who had complained that the operation made her less of a woman. It developed that Nora had insisted that Eddie use condoms ever since she found out that genital warts might have been a factor in causing her cancer. She believed, with good reason, that Eddie was chronically unfaithful, and she has found bills from massage parlors in his pockets.

Eddie had left Nora several times, claiming that she was the unfaithful one. He detests condoms and has said he cannot enjoy intercourse when wearing one. He also complained that Nora's vagina is too shallow, but the psychologist thought this was probably a convenient way to score more points in the psychological warfare with his wife. Nora and Eddie did not want to divorce because she was dependent on his medical insurance and he did not want to lose their house or disrupt the lives of their teenaged children. They will probably continue to torment each other until death doth them part.

The Average Guys

Most couples do have reasonable sexual communication. Over their years together, they might have established a lovemaking routine that is satisfying to both partners. Occasionally, one might ask to try something a little different. Although initiating sex often is largely one partner's role, at times the other might give signals of being in the mood. Sex is not the most important element of the couple's relationship, but it is a comforting part of their bond.

If cancer disrupts the average couple's sex life, however, their typical sexual communication might not be adequate to openly confront the new problems.

Eva, aged 42, and her husband had both been happy with their sex life before her treatment for breast cancer interfered. Sex happened without effort or thought. They rarely talked about their lovemaking in detail, but they did spend a good deal of time kissing and touching. Oral and manual caressing were routine for them, and they had several favorite positions for intercourse. Eva had been warned that her chemotherapy would make her menopausal, and she already was experiencing annoying hot flashes. To minimize vaginal dryness, she used a gel lubricant the first time she and her husband tried sex. To her shock, however, Eva had great difficulty getting aroused. When her husband caressed her breasts, her only thought was about breast cancer. When he brushed his hand over her belly, she felt the soreness of her scar from breast reconstruction. She wanted the light off so that he would not see her without pubic hair and with only one nipple. After a long time of caressing, she signaled him to go ahead and try penetration. Even with the lubricant, Eva's vagina felt dry and tight. Thrusting hurt. She tried to hide her feelings, but tears dripped out of her eyes and her husband stopped. He held her while she sobbed. "I don't think I'll ever be normal again," she gasped. "What are we going to do?" He tried to reassure her that he loved her and would live without sex until she felt more ready.

After that night, Eva's husband did not bring up the topic of sex. He still cuddled with his wife and, indeed, made an extra effort to give her compliments and tell her how much he loved her. He wanted to wait to try sex again until she felt ready. He was horrified at the idea of hurting her physically. Because he did not communicate these thoughts to Eva, however, she feared that he was no longer attracted to her. Even as she felt better, she was reluctant to initiate sex. What if her husband just went along because he felt sorry for her? What if they tried and he could not even get an erection because she was so ugly? What if intercourse still hurt as much as it had the first time?

Eva and her husband needed some outside advice and help to make a new effort with sex. Their first failure had been so traumatic that neither partner felt confident about trying again. Ironically, their lack of communication was really due to their fear of hurting each other's feelings. The net result, however, was that they went for months without any sexual contact before a visit to Eva's oncologist and a referral for sexual counseling broke the impasse.

Sexual Athletes

A smaller group of men and women describe sex lives like the ones on TV talk shows. Sex is a central pleasure in their lives, and any loss of capacity or attractiveness is as devastating as a medical handicap would be to a star athlete. Their ability to talk explicitly about sex is not the issue. But though they may have exchanged vivid sexual fantasies or played erotic games, talking about a sexual problem to a partner can be very threatening.

Jerrod, a 24-year-old law student, had operations to remove one testicle and the lymph node drainage system as treatment for testicular cancer. Some men no longer ejaculate semen after this surgery, but Jerrod's surgeon had been able to spare nerves to preserve his fertility. Nevertheless, Jerrod was angry at the world. "Look at the length of this scar!" he complained, pulling up his polo shirt to reveal a well-muscled torso. "How am I going to explain that to a girl?" My hair hides most of the scar on my sac, but this looks like I was split in two! I don't even feel comfortable with my shirt off in public. I haven't been swimming since my operation, and I used to go three times a week."

Jerrod also noticed that he had less semen at ejaculation and felt it no longer spurted out strongly. "It kind of drips out now," he said. He was not worried about his fertility over the next several years, but he was afraid a partner might feel his orgasm was abnormal, especially with intercourse. "Girls always tell me they feel me come inside of them," he said. "That's why I don't like to use rubbers." Jerrod was scornful of the psychologist's suggestion that most women do not actually feel semen spurting into their vaginas during intercourse.

Jerrod did not have a steady dating partner, but typically dated several different women. An evening at his favorite night spot often ended in casual sex with a new partner. Jerrod was proud of his ability to ask women to try all kinds of sexual positions or to act out fantasies with him. He felt stigmatized by his cancer, however, and did not look forward to answering women's questions about his scars. "I think I'll just say I had a hernia," he mused.

Opening Up Communication about Sex

No matter what your style of sexual communication has been, if you want to communicate openly with your partner about cancer and your sexuality, here are some guidelines to make the process more comfortable.

Create a Safe Space and Time

Whether you have been married for thirty years or are dating someone new, it is usually easier to discuss sex outside of the bedroom. An "Ahem . . ." while you are lying naked on the bed in a hotel honeymoon suite after three vacation nights without any sex is not a good opening for a relaxed talk. Choose a time when you are not exhausted or stressed out.

Talking during sex can be distracting. Sexual excitement involves intense concentration, similar to a trance state. To stay aroused, you need to focus your attention on pleasurable physical sensations or erotic mental images. You can shift your concentration momentarily to guide your partner's touch or to respond to a request and then return to your building sensations; but taking time out to have a major conversation might really break the mood.

Just after lovemaking, you might feel sleepy instead of alert. A discussion after sex can also resemble instant replays on a sports show. Instead of analyzing what just went wrong, it is better to plan ahead to make the next time a success.

Make sure you will not be interrupted by kids or phone calls. If you pick a public place to talk about sex, find one that gives you enough privacy to avoid embarrassment, for example, a quiet restaurant with widely spaced tables or a beach at sunset. A tête-à-tête in the front seat of the car with your toddlers fighting in the rear does not qualify.

If you are starting a new sexual relationship, you might have some unsettling information to tell your partner, for example, that you have a urinary ostomy, are infertile, or can no longer get firm erections. (Chapter 28 focuses on the special concerns of single people.) In general, it is easiest to wait to discuss your cancer until you feel that a new partner is becoming a trustworthy friend. On the other hand, you do not want to postpone your talk until you are taking off your clothes together or, worse yet, until your wedding night.

Choose One or Two Goals

It is easiest to improve your sex life if you can focus on one or two goals at a time. If you tell your partner that your whole sex life is a disaster, the two of you will be at a loss to know where to start in making things better. Ask your partner to work with you on putting more fun back into your sex life. You can talk together about ways to be more playful or relaxed. The more specific your goals are, the better.

> Martha and Josh had only tried sex two or three times in the year since his bone marrow transplant for leukemia. Josh was having trouble keeping his erections. When sex did not go well, he was in a bad mood for several days. Finally, Martha told her husband how much she missed their sex life. They agreed to try more often, but another two months went by without any lovemaking. At New Year's, Martha told Josh she was making a resolution to initiate some kind of sexual touching at least twice a month. "I don't care if it ends in intercourse," she said, "but I want us to feel close again." Martha kept her promise, and sexual touching became more frequent and pleasurable. Josh's erections were still poor, however. He told his wife he would follow her example and set himself a small, weekly goal related to sex. The first week he found out where he could go for help for his erection problem. The next week he made an appointment. Long before the next New Year, Josh and Martha were enjoying intercourse.

After one partner has suggested a goal, it is important to make sure the other partner is in tune. Perhaps a wife thinks that the way to get comfortable with sex after her mastectomy is to wear her breast prosthesis with sexy lingerie that covers her breast area. She does not want her husband to touch either of her breasts because she does not want to be reminded during sex of her cancer. Her husband thinks they should have sex totally in the nude, as they always did in the past. He wants to feel free to caress not only his wife's remaining breast, but the scar from her surgery. He sees this approach as being more honest and thinks it would help his wife overcome her fears about her breast cancer. Both styles of coping can work, and neither partner is right or wrong. If they do not discuss their opposing views, however, and reach some consensus, they will probably each end up quite frustrated.

Focus on the Positive

It is crucial to define your goals in positive terms. If you tell your wife, "I'm sick and tired of you lying there passively the whole time we have sex," she will probably feel hurt and angry. If you say, "I would really like you to caress me more actively during sex, especially now that my illness has made it hard to get excited," she is much more likely to hear you and give it a try.

Remember that sexual communication is an ongoing process. Perhaps you feel that you have told your partner many times what you want during sex, but he or she always seems to forget. Over time, you have become frustrated and angry and feel it is just not worth it to try communicating again. Perhaps you need to guide your partner's hand a few times during lovemaking itself or to use short, upbeat suggestions during sex; for example, "That's the right place, but I need a lighter touch," or "That feels so good, please don't stop yet," or "I'm enjoying foreplay so much, I'm not quite ready for intercourse."

Avoid Arguments

Perhaps sex has always been a loaded subject in your relationship. If you worry that a conversation about resuming sex could degenerate into bickering, begin by setting some guidelines with your partner: "I feel very sensitive to rejection, and I also worry about hurting your feelings. Let's try to talk about our sex life without getting defensive. Let's agree to be gentle and positive when we make suggestions to each other about changing our sex life. We can stop this talk at any time if one of us is starting to feel hurt or upset."

Discuss Your Fear of Sexual Rejection

If your cancer treatment has affected your appearance or your ability to function sexually, your worst fear might be that your partner will reject you because of the changes. Although disclosing your insecurity can be painful, telling your partner directly about your fear often clears the air. Try to trust that your partner is also responding honestly. Suppose a wife says that her husband's erection problem does not bother her much. She has always enjoyed sexual caressing more than penetration, anyway. In my experience, the man often doubts that she is telling the truth, fearing she is just trying to reassure him. Men commonly feel so terrible about an erection problem that they urge their wives or girlfriends to leave and find someone who can satisfy them sexually. The usual result of this noble speech is a very indignant and frustrated woman.

Women tend to worry about physical scars or ostomy appliances. Rather than expressing their fears, they often avoid sex by undressing in the closet or coming to bed so late that their mates have fallen asleep. Ostomies or scars are usually much more devastating to the person who has them than they are to the partner, however. On the other hand, perhaps your partner is having difficulty accepting the physical changes caused by your disease. Even though such feedback is very painful, you need to listen and try to find solutions. If your partner cannot accept you after cancer, consider seeking help from a mental health professional.

Discuss Your Fears about Breaking Up

Most couples find that cancer strengthens their commitment. In a shaky relationship, however, illness can indeed be the straw that breaks the camel's back. If you feel your relationship is in danger, it is better to discuss the situation openly than to pretend that everything is fine.

Jack left his wife when he was 54 and fell in love with Amanda, a 29-year-old junior executive at the company where he was a vice president. Their relationship was common knowledge at the office, leading to a great deal of gossip and even some threat to their jobs. Just a few months into the divorce negotiations, Jack was diagnosed with prostate cancer and had a radical prostatectomy.

Amanda visited in the hospital, but Jack's estranged wife and young adult children also were very much involved in supporting him through his illness. His wife saw the cancer as a possible opening for a reconciliation. Jack was grateful for her concern, but he found himself obsessing about whether Amanda would still want to marry him. His surgeon assured him that he had an excellent chance of recovering good erections, and Jack knew he could use a medical or surgical treatment to restore erections if needed. He was more upset over becoming infertile. Because of Jack's age, the surgeon had not emphasized fertility before surgery, and Jack was very angry that he had not been given a chance to bank sperm. He knew Amanda wanted children, and now he could not be their biological father unless the couple went through the expense and risk of in vitro fertilization. He also had difficulty coping with the temporary incontinence he experienced during his recovery. From being a fit and powerful executive who looked younger than his years, he felt he had become a dependent invalid, less than a full man.

Jack was never one to hide his feelings, and he and Amanda had several major arguments even before he left the hospital. She was very threatened by Jack's wife's involvement in his care and believed Jack should have banished his wife from the hospital. Jack wanted Amanda to move into his condo temporarily to help him when he went home from the hospital. She refused, saying that they had already had enough trouble at work without openly living together. He accused her of caring more for her career than for him. Jack was afraid to tell Amanda about his infertility, but in the end he explained it all to her. He offered to set her free from their engagement. Amanda decided she did not want to marry Jack. In fact, she found a job in another state. Jack eventually moved back into his marriage.

For childless couples who had planned to start a family, infertility after cancer might sometimes precipitate a divorce. If a couple is not yet married at the time of cancer diagnosis, the anticipated difficulties in having children can affect partners' readiness to commit to each other. This is another situation in which some professional counseling might help partners clarify their feelings.

If you sense unspoken fears that cancer is alienating you from your partner, perhaps you need to declare your own love and commitment more openly.

Guy and his wife had not tried any sexual touching since he began his interferon therapy for chronic leukemia. He was still feeling tired; but he was back to work full time, and life, for the most part, had returned to normal. He knew he eventually would probably need a bone marrow transplant, but he tried not to think about it. Sometimes he could forget his disease for hours at a time. Guy's leukemia made him reevaluate his priorities. He wanted to spend time with his family, take more vacations, and savor each day. His desire for sex had dropped noticeably since his diagnosis, however, and he could tell that his wife was upset.

Finally he planned an evening when the couple went out for a quiet dinner. Their daughter was staying overnight with a friend. When they got home, Guy turned on the gas fireplace and asked his wife to sit with him on the couch. "Going through this illness really has reminded me how much I love you and value your support. I think our marriage has always been good, but sometimes we've taken each other for granted. I think I often don't tell you how I feel, and I just wanted you to know how important you are to me."

Guy's wife hugged him tight. She didn't say anything, and he realized that she was trying not to cry. The couple just held each other for several minutes. Guy told his wife that he had been afraid to try sex for fear he would be unable to satisfy her. This conversation cleared the air and helped the couple to begin sexual activity without expecting everything to go smoothly.

Discuss Your Fears about Survival and Recurrence

Some couples put sex on hold because they become overwhelmed by the fear of dying from cancer. It is hard to get in the mood for sex if you are seeing life as one long good-bye. A more helpful perspective is to get the most out of each day. You might die of cancer in two years or two months— or you might get mowed down tomorrow by a drunken driver. Why not affirm life by enjoying sex in the meanwhile?

Susan's husband had Hodgkin's disease. The couple was in their late twenties and had a baby boy when Larry began chemotherapy. The treatment was successful, but after a year of remission, Larry's cancer reoccurred. During the months of his second round of treatments, Susan often had nightmares about being at her husband's funeral. She had been working as a kindergarten teacher until her pregnancy, but the couple had planned their finances so that she would be able to stay home while their children were young. Now there would probably never be a second child for them. She often cried in secret when she thought of her son growing up without his father, but, most of all, she hated the thought of losing her own lover and best friend.

Even when Larry was grouchy and depressed during his treatment, Susan rarely felt annoyed at him. She did not flinch at emptying his vomit tray or learning to give him injections. She just wanted him around. When Larry was too ill to have sex, Susan rarely felt frustrated. She did cuddle close to Larry whenever she could, and, on his good days, they made sure to take time for sex. They even discussed his wish that she have a happy life without guilt if he died. Susan knew she would go on, because she had her son who needed her. These thoughts did not ease her pain much, but they did help her cope with her daily fear of losing Larry.

Be a Good Listener

After a successful talk about sex, both partners should feel they really got their points across. It is a good idea to summarize your partner's requests for changes and goals out loud. Ask if you heard your partner correctly. Check out the messages your partner received from what you said.

Now that you have some good ideas about how to express your sexual feelings and concerns, you are ready to think about taking steps to resume a more active sex life.

5

Going Back to Bed

Cancer treatment is usually followed by a period during which you are unable to have sex. That period could be as short as a week or two after surgery or as long as several months during and after a bone marrow transplant. At the appropriate time, the doctor might tell you in a matter-of-fact tone that you can resume your sex life (although more commonly she never mentions the topic of sex). Facing that first try at sex can be so anxiety-provoking, however, that many men or women put it off for weeks, months, or forever.

This chapter suggests how to set up a sexual situation to maximize enjoyment and minimize disappointment. The first step is usually the toughest. Start small and savor your successes.

Rethinking the Performance Model of Sex

Our society promotes the idea that sex is a performance. Sexual people are young, healthy, thin, and beautiful. They fall into each other's arms, gasping with passion, regardless of the time of day or surroundings. After a few seconds of kissing, or perhaps a brief interlude of oral sex, the man has a powerful erection. The woman has multiple orgasms the moment penetration takes place. After twenty or thirty minutes of thrusting, with several changes of position, the couple might snooze for a few minutes before starting the whole process again.

In the performance model of sex, a woman never needs to decide whether to wear her wig for lovemaking. A man never has an ostomy appliance that comes unglued and leaks urine during intercourse. Nobody is ever tired or nauseated when a partner wants to have sex. Sweet nothings are never whispered with a speech aid and erections never need some extra help. Lovers never have a missing leg or a facial scar.

How much of the performance model has crept into your expectations about sex? How can you give yourself more room to enjoy sex in the real world? Try this exercise in changing your perspective: Think about your-self before your cancer. What were your top three assets as a lover? Think about yourself today. What are your top three assets as a lover now? If you believe you lost some important quality as a result of your cancer, have you gained something else valuable? For example, you might have lost the ability to have firm erections, but perhaps you have become expert at bringing your partner to orgasm with oral sex.

Finding Time for Sex: The Minivacation

One of the thorniest problems of modern life is finding time for sex. Lovers often put a low priority on time to talk, enjoy a mutually pleasurable non-sexual activity (other than watching TV), and feel close. Without private time, many people find themselves feeling alienated or unattracted to their partner.

Especially if sex has become problematic, couples often propose taking a romantic vacation to make time for each other. This sounds like a great idea, but often is not too practical. Vacations take time and money that might not be available. There might not be anyone to look after the kids, pets, or house. If one partner is still ill, it might not be a good idea to risk being far from the medical team.

Another problem with using a vacation to improve your sex life is that it creates a pressure situation. If you have the penthouse suite complete with mirrored bed and sex is still a disaster, you might feel even worse than you did at home (plus you ruin your vacation).

A better idea is to schedule minivacations every few days—an evening or afternoon when your first priority is private leisure time as a couple. If you still have children at home, finding and affording a baby-sitter can be a problem. Perhaps your vacation will only be an hour or two after the kids are asleep. Try starting out with some transition time to put aside the cares of your daily life—even if that only means a half hour to recline in a bubble bath or read a novel.

The setting also contributes to the mood. To set this special time apart, try to find a place and time where you will not be interrupted. Take the phone off the hook, or perhaps turn on your answering machine. One of you can take responsibility for making the room comfortable. Try to avoid places that are too hot or cold. If possible, put on some music that you both enjoy to help you shut out the outside world. Soft lighting is helpful, especially if one of you feels self-conscious about appearance.

Rediscovering the Joys of "Petting"

Some people are physically unable to have intercourse after their cancer treatment; for example, a man might no longer get firm erections, or a woman might experience severe pain with penetration. Yet many older couples, in particular, have never brought each other to orgasm through hand or oral caressing and are reluctant to experiment. Gay couples have an advantage here because they typically enjoy a wide variety of lovemaking techniques.

Was there a time in your sex life when sex meant "making out"? Most young adults explore sexual sensations through kissing and caressing, often with most of their clothes on. Although those first experiences can be frustrating or even frightening, they also are often very pleasurable. Although most people think of intercourse as "grown-up" sex, many teenagers find it a disappointment, compared with the thrill of petting.

If you have discontinued intercourse or genital caressing because of your cancer treatment, a first step to enjoying sex again is to rediscover making out. Ask your partner to make a solemn agreement just to stop at kissing on the couch, caressing each other with all your clothes on, or perhaps exchanging orgasms through hand caressing. The idea is to have fun without worrying about failing.

Jane had a tumor of the spinal cord when she was in her late teens. Although surgery and radiation therapy successfully controlled the cancer, she was left in a wheelchair, with loss of movement and sensation from her waist down. Jane had already been engaged to Brad and sexually active when her cancer was diagnosed. When she returned to college, the couple agreed that they would begin by just kissing. Their tentative kisses soon became more passionate. They also exchanged back rubs. Jane could sit up against pillows and reach Brad's back. She still had sensation over her upper back and could experience sensual pleasure from Brad's touch. At first Jane was afraid to let Brad see her nude. She was sad that her legs had become wasted from the paralysis. Brad reassured Jane that he still found her beautiful. Now that her genital area had little feeling, she learned how to reach orgasm from breast caressing and kissing.

Rub-a-Dub-Dub: Start Out in the Tub

Many people find water a relaxing environment. If you are feeling anxious about sexual touching, consider a sensual shower with a partner as a first step. You can use scented soap or shower gel to caress each other's bodies. Big bathtubs or hot tubs also lend themselves to playfulness. Some bubble bath, romantic music, or candlelight can help to set the mood.

Nate did not regard himself as a vain man. At age 69, he had already coped with a receding hairline, some extra pounds, and many wrinkles. When he had surgery to remove his bladder and had to wear an ostomy pouch to collect his urine, however, Nate found himself very self-conscious. He had several incidents in the first weeks at home when his ostomy pouch leaked. Once he was playing golf and had to hurry back to the locker room to change. He was very worried about smelling like urine, although his wife, Letty, told him he was fine. Nate and Letty had only been married for two years, and, because his wife was ten years younger, Nate obsessed about keeping up with their active lifestyle.

Nate's urologist suggested he use penile injections to get firmer erections after surgery. In a special office visit, Nate was instructed on using injections and given medication to take home. Still, over the next two weeks, he did not initiate sex. He finally told Letty that he was horrified by the thought that his ostomy bag would come unglued during sex and that he would leak urine all over. Letty was reassuring, "Remember, dear, that the doctor said urine is sterile. It may not smell good, but it wouldn't hurt either one of us."

That night, after Nate was already in his pajamas, Letty came into the bedroom wearing one of her prettiest robes. Instead of getting in bed, she asked her husband to come into the bathroom. She had the water already running in their large shower and had put scented soap and a big loofah sponge inside. Letty unbuttoned her husband's pajamas and asked him to take off her robe. "Come on in," she invited him, holding open the shower door. "The water's fine; and if you spring a leak, we'll never know the difference."

Dancing the Fright Away

Dance is a universal human pleasure, and one that is associated with courtship and sex in most cultures. When you are trying to get more sexual after cancer, dancing to your favorite music can help to build a romantic or sexual mood. Sexy dancing can take many forms—partners holding each other close and swaying slowly, prancing to rock music, ballroom dancing, folk dancing, or even aerobic dancing! The physical exercise helps increase your pulse and deepen your breathing—cues that feel a lot like sexual excitement.

> David was divorced when his lymphoma was diagnosed. He had a casual dating relationship that broke up during his chemotherapy. After he finished his treatments and his hair grew back, David felt lonely and sexually frustrated. He was reluctant to ask women out. When would he tell them about his cancer? Would any woman want to have a relationship with him if she knew? A buddy persuaded David to go with him to a singles dance. As the evening wore on, David relaxed and found that women came up and asked him to dance. During a slow song, he held an attractive partner close and found himself getting an erection. The woman did not seem to mind and, in fact, leaned closer. For the first time since his cancer, David could imagine having a sexual relationship again.

Flying Solo

Experimenting with self-touch can be a reassuring and helpful way to resume sex after cancer. When you touch your own body, you can focus on the sensations you feel without worrying about your partner's pleasure. Your body gives you immediate feedback, guiding you how and where to touch. If masturbation gives you pleasurable feelings, helps you get an erection, or allows you to reach an orgasm, you know that your sexual response is still in working order. If you discover that caressing feels different, you can teach your partner how to alter the way that he or she touches you. For men and women who do not have a sexual partner, masturbation is an opportunity to explore sexual capacity and soothe sexual frustration after cancer treatment.

Although as many as 90 percent of American men and 60 percent of women try masturbation during their lifetimes, it is still a taboo topic in our society. Contrary to the stereotype that solitary masturbation replaces the need for a partner, a recent survey found that people who have frequent sex lives with their spouses are also those most likely to masturbate regularly. (For more positive thoughts on masturbation, see *The New Male Sexuality* in Resources under Books.) Research has also shown that women who masturbate to orgasm are more likely to reach orgasm regularly during intercourse.

Perhaps you believe from a religious standpoint that masturbation is wrong. Many organized religions frown on masturbation because it gives sexual pleasure but does not lead to reproduction. Perhaps if people masturbate, they might also succumb to other temptations, such as having sex with a partner outside of marriage. Spirituality is an important aspect of life, and I would not challenge anyone to change his or her religious values. However, you might also have heard that masturbation is unhealthy from a medical standpoint or is an activity that promotes homosexuality. There is no scientific evidence for either of these ideas. If masturbation is repugnant to you personally, however, trying it is unlikely to be helpful.

Sensate Focus: A Framework for Exploring Sexual Touch

A series of three exercises in intimate touch can provide a framework for resuming sex in a relaxed, nonpressured way. These exercises were named "sensate focus" by Masters and Johnson, the originators of sex therapy in the 1960s. The idea is to focus on your sensual pleasure, without expecting to get sexually aroused at first. In *Step 1* of the exercise, partners spend a whole hour exchanging body caresses without including breast or genital touch. In *Step 2*, there is some brief, exploring sexual touch, but not to the point of orgasm. In *Step 3*, the person being touched has the option to ask the partner to continue hand caressing to the point of orgasm.

Getting Started

Busy couples often find that they need to plan ahead, making a date to do the exercise together. You and your partner might want to take turns in initiating the exercise. If you are comfortable with nudity, it leaves all areas of your body free for caressing. Sensate focus exercises provide a way to get used to having your partner see and touch areas of your body affected by cancer treatment. For example, a woman who has had breast reconstruction might want to start out by covering the area with a pretty bra or camisole. Gradually she could get more comfortable with uncovering her breasts and then with trying some light touching of that area. Some couples enjoy rubbing scented body oils into each other's skin as part of the touching.

It is almost always best to start with Step 1. If you and your partner find the exercise very relaxing and enjoyable, you can go on to Step 2 the next time. Otherwise, you might want to repeat Step 1 until you feel you have gotten the most out of it. You can handle the transition from Step 2 to Step 3 in the same way.

If your attempts to have sex have been frustrating and have made you feel like a failure, you and your partner might wish to limit your lovemaking to sensate focus touch until you successfully complete all three exercises. If you want to continue more traditional lovemaking, save it for a separate occasion. Sensate focus exercises work best when you know that there is no performance pressure. It is hard to stay relaxed if, at the back of your mind, you anticipate having "real sex" if the sensate focus touch goes well.

Step 1:   In this exercise, partners take turns being the *giver* and *receiver* of touch. It does not matter who goes first. When you are the receiver, lie on your stomach. The giver spends at least fifteen minutes touching the back of your body. Then you turn over for fifteen minutes of touching your front side. The amount of time is just a guideline, but remember that it is easy to skimp on time during the touch. Then you might not get enough practice in mental focusing.

In Step 1, the giver does not touch the receiver's breast or genital areas. Touch is limited in this way to reduce any psychological pressure to feel sexually excited. Instead, the receiver's job is to tune into the bodily feelings he or she experiences while being caressed. It might take five or ten minutes just to let go of thoughts about disliking your body, boring your partner, or feeling guilty about household chores that you left undone. Each time you catch yourself thinking about something other than your physical reaction to the touch, remind yourself to focus on your sensations. This type of focusing is a skill, similar to meditation. Think of your attention like a camera lens. You are bringing your skin sensations into sharp focus, letting all other thoughts and feelings fuzz out.

As giver, too, focus on the pleasure you experience from touching and caressing. Notice what you like about your partner's body—the smooth shapes or soft skin that you enjoy touching. Be creative in varying your touch. Include as many parts of your partner's body as you can (except for the breasts and genitals). Some touch can include sensual massage, but other caressing can be light and teasing. You can touch your partner with your hair or with your hand, or you can add in occasional kisses. Try not to worry about supplying the kinds of caresses you know your partner likes the best. Your job is to explore a variety of kinds of touch and to enjoy your role as giver.

As receiver, do not talk much. If you ooh and aah to signal the giver about your likes and dislikes, you might distract yourself from focusing on sensation. If the giver uses a touch that tickles or feels unpleasant, speak up, however. Try to give your feedback in the form of a positive request: "I like it when you touch my feet, but that light touch tickles. How about more of a slow massage?" Feeling ticklish is a common problem the first time you try the exercise, but that usually decreases as you become more relaxed.

When you have had your thirty-minute turn as receiver, take a break and tell your partner three specific types of touch that you enjoyed the most. Be as explicit in describing the touch as possible so that your partner would be able to touch you the same way again. For example, "I really liked it when you ran your palm very lightly down the center of my back." This kind of detailed feedback is good practice for later steps, when you guide your partner in caressing your genital areas. It is usually more difficult to state your preferences for genital touch as clearly. You can also tell your partner one touch that you liked the least. Keep the main focus on the positive, however.

In the second half of the exercise, switch roles. The giver becomes the receiver and vice versa. Again, take a couple of minutes afterward to give verbal feedback about the touches that felt especially pleasurable. If one or both of you feel some sexual excitement, enjoy the pleasure. Getting aroused is not a measure of the success of the exercise, however. Rather, the goals are to decrease feelings of self-consciousness and to increase your sense of relaxation and intimacy during touch.

Occasionally, one partner finds the sensate focus exercise upsetting. Lying still and being touched might bring up bad memories of forced sexual touch in the past; for example, if a person had been raped or molested. More commonly, one partner feels awkward about doing the exercise instead of having traditional sex. Sometimes people who are chronically tense and pressured about time have great trouble relaxing and focusing on the touch. Occasionally, one partner feels unbearably frustrated by touch that does not lead to orgasms or intercourse. If the exercise brings up negative feelings, you might want to seek help from a mental health professional trained in sex therapy (see Resources under Information Networks).

Step 2:   Step 2 follows the same framework as Step 1—taking the giver and receiver roles and spending an hour on sensual touch. The main difference in Step 2 is that the giver can touch any part of the receiver's body, including the breast and genital areas. Caressing of those more sexual parts of the body should make up only a brief part of the overall exercise, however, and should include only light and exploring touch. Touching to the point of orgasm is still not included. Step 2 gives you a chance to enjoy genital caressing without expecting it to be highly sexually exciting. It does not matter whether or not you have erections or vaginal lubrication.

One other change is that the receiver can guide the giver more directly during the exercise, either by explaining in words the kind of touch you prefer or by guiding the giver's hand. You can put your hand over your partner's to demonstrate exactly the type of touch that would give you pleasure, or you can touch yourself, with the giver's hand riding piggyback on yours. Then the giver can see and feel exactly how you like to be touched. Guiding a partner's hand is especially helpful with genital caressing because it is often difficult to explain your desires in words.

Step 3:   Step 3 is exactly like Steps 1 and 2, except that more of the time can be devoted to caressing the breasts and genital areas. As the receiver, you can ask the giver to prolong the sexual touching until you have an orgasm. If you are not in the mood to try for an orgasm or if you feel like the touching has gone on long enough, you can also choose to stop. The goal of the exercise is still pleasure, rather than reaching orgasm.

If both partners in a couple are comfortable with oral sex, you can include it in Step 3. If you are a man with an erection problem, you might get anxious during Step 3 if your penis does not become or stay hard. One way to avoid focusing on performance is to have the giver deliberately stop caressing your penis if you get a firm erection, allowing your erection to fade. The giver can focus on other kinds of pleasurable touch, only returning to your penis after several minutes. If you get an erection again, focus touch away from your penis a second time. After two tries at getting and losing erections, the giver can go on to bring you to orgasm.

Some couples avoid having the man ejaculate outside the woman's vagina because they feel uncomfortable with semen. Semen is often viewed as dirty or disgusting. Men worry that a partner will be turned off by seeing them ejaculate. Women often do not like the smell or taste of semen. It might help to think of semen as a fluid very similar to egg white in color and texture. It contains the sperm cells and chemicals that help them stay lively and healthy during reproduction. If you feel a bit anxious about semen, try keeping some tissues or a damp washcloth by the bed.

Coping with Physical Symptoms

During and after cancer treatment, you might have periods of chronic fatigue, nausea, or pain. It is difficult to get in the mood for sex if you feel miserable. On the other hand, if your symptoms are relatively mild, a relaxed and sensual session of lovemaking might help to distract you from feeling ill.

One key to staying sexually active despite an illness is giving up some spontaneity in scheduling sex. Try having sex during your good periods; for example, at the time of day when you feel most rested and when your pain medication is in effect, or in the few days just before a round of chemotherapy when you have recovered from many side effects of the last course.

You might need to prepare for sex. Maybe you need to take pain medication at a certain time before the hour when you plan to make love. If you are self-catheterizing your bladder or have a urinary ostomy, take care to empty your system of urine before sex. If you are struggling with joint stiffness, take a warm bath before you get into bed with your partner.

If you are quite ill, you might need to redefine your sex life. Perhaps you just are not up to having vigorous intercourse, but you long for cuddling, or you would enjoy being able to lie back while your partner brought you to orgasm through oral sex. Discuss your needs and limitations openly with your partner.

Most people do achieve satisfying sex lives after their cancer treatment. Although we have focused on the positive, it is also important to be aware of ways to prevent unwanted side effects of sex: sexually transmitted diseases and unintended pregnancy.

6

Safer Sex after Cancer: Preventing Disease and Unwanted Pregnancy

So far, we have talked about how to preserve your sex life during and after cancer treatment—but you might be worried about whether it is really safe to have sex.

Does Cancer Ever Make Sex Unsafe?

Your physician might temporarily ban sex in a few medical situations. If your immune system is very severely depressed, for example, during chemotherapy, you might need to avoid sexual contact (as well as other close encounters). If a tumor in your bladder, cervix, or rectal area is bleeding heavily, you might be asked to skip sex until cancer treatment has decreased the risk of triggering a hemorrhage. If you had surgery, there could be a period of several weeks during which a variety of daily life activities, including sex, might be too strenuous.

In most other situations, it is safe to stay sexually active during and after cancer treatment. As I already mentioned, cancer is not contagious through sexual activity. Having sex has no known influence on whether cancer returns or progresses.

Some chemotherapy drugs make their way into semen or vaginal fluids and have been linked to genital irritation in a patient's sexual partner. No clear guidelines are available, but it makes sense to use condoms for oral sex or intercourse during chemotherapy. At least in theory, condom use could be especially important for a pregnant woman whose husband is on chemotherapy. Many drugs can cause birth defects, especially early in pregnancy when a woman might not even be aware of her condition. To my knowledge, no case of a miscarriage or birth defect has ever been linked to a woman's exposure to chemotherapy from sexual activity with her partner. Given the small amounts of drug present in semen, there is a very low risk that a developing fetus would be exposed to these chemicals. But why take a chance?

Times to Avoid Pregnancy

When men or women are told they will be infertile after cancer treatment, they might assume they no longer need to use contraception. If you are not ready for a baby, do not count on being infertile unless you are sure your cancer treatment made pregnancy permanently impossible. Men often regain fertility after chemotherapy or lower doses of radiation therapy and even sometimes after a bone marrow transplant. Women can still be fertile even if their periods have stopped or have been irregular for several months.

Remember that pregnancy can occur during radiation therapy or chemotherapy in young women or in the wives of men undergoing treatment. To avoid any risk of birth defects, it is wise to prevent pregnancy during cancer treatment. If you cannot find an acceptable type of contraception, you should stop having intercourse.

But if a pregnancy does develop during one partner's cancer treatment, do not panic. Despite concerns about the impact of chemotherapy or radiation, the rate of birth defects after exposure to cancer treatment in babies who are carried successfully to term is not unusually high (see Chapter 21).

During Chemotherapy for Men

Most chemotherapy drugs do not destroy sperm cell production until a certain dose has been given. Some drugs might not decrease sperm production at all, but they could potentially damage the genetic material of developing sperm cells. The risk of birth defects in children conceived with sperm cells exposed to chemotherapy is unknown. The safest choice is to use contraception once chemotherapy begins and continue using it until three months after the end of treatment, when any exposed sperm cells should be "used up."

During Radiation Therapy for Men

Men who receive radiation therapy also do not become infertile right away. Sperm cells that are already ripe or close to ripe are resistant to radiation and unlikely to be damaged in the early days of radiation therapy. Sperm cells are more fragile in their early stages, however, and their genetic material could be damaged, especially by radiation aimed near the testicles. To minimize the chance of conceiving a child with a damaged sperm cell, a man could take steps to prevent pregnancy from the time he begins radiation therapy until three months have passed since the end of treatment. A man does not transmit radiation to his partner, so a couple could use any type of effective contraception they prefer.

During Radiation Therapy in Women

A woman who is going to start radiation should make sure to prevent a pregnancy because the developing fetus is highly sensitive to radiation damage. If a woman has radiation therapy aimed at her pelvis or abdomen early in pregnancy, she usually will miscarry. Even later in pregnancy, radiation exposure can cause birth defects.

During Chemotherapy in Women

A woman might remain fertile during chemotherapy, even if her menstrual cycles become irregular or stop. She should still consult her physician about using effective contraception during chemotherapy or should avoid sexual activity. The risk of damage to fetal development during early pregnancy from chemotherapy is high. Women often miscarry spontaneously. If chemotherapy becomes necessary later in pregnancy, especially the third trimester, it is not as dangerous to the fetus, although the baby could still be born prematurely or with low birth weight.

Cancer and Sexually Transmitted Diseases

A variety of sexually transmitted diseases (STDs) have become common in our society. Most young people today will have several sexual partners across their lifetimes. Not only is the pill a very effective means of birth control, but it has reduced the popularity of barrier contraceptives, like condoms and diaphragms, that can prevent the spread of STDs. The ease of traveling across the globe has also helped spread STDs from one end of the earth to the other. The human immunodeficiency virus (HIV) is one of the deadliest STDs, but it is also one of the least common. Lesser known germs, such as the human papilloma virus (HPV) and chlamydia, contribute to cancer risk or infertility, but they get less publicity.

STDs Can Promote Cancer

A few STDs can increase cancer risk. HPV normally causes painless growths in the genital area in men or women, but some strains of HPV promote cancer of the anus, cervix, vulva, or penis. The immune system can fight back against HPV-related changes. But in a person whose immune system is suppressed for a long period (e.g., the person has HIV, uses drugs to inactivate the immune system after an organ transplant, or has months of chemotherapy), HPV has more chance to promote cancer. Women who have had a kidney, liver, or heart transplant have a tenfold increased risk of cancer of the cervix or vulva. Tobacco use also gives HPV more free reign.

One of the lethal outcomes of HIV infection is cancer, especially Kaposi's sarcoma (mainly seen in gay men), non-Hodgkin's lymphoma, and squamous cell cancers of the anus and cervix.

STDs Can Flare Up during Cancer Treatment

If you have ever been diagnosed with HIV, genital herpes, or genital warts (HPV), you might want to alert your oncologist before you begin a cancer therapy that depresses the immune system. During chemotherapy (especially a bone marrow transplant) or even radiotherapy, an infection such as genital herpes can turn from a mild annoyance to a very painful and sometimes dangerous complication of treatment. Medications might prevent a severe outbreak during your treatment; for example, the drug acyclovir (Zovirax) can prevent or shorten herpes symptoms.

How to Have Safer Sex

If you have never had an STD, you certainly do not want to get one now! If you are sexually active, unless you have a long-term, monogamous relationship with a partner you can trust completely, you should practice safer sex. Notice I say *safer*. There is no guaranteed safe sex. The most effective protection against STDs is condoms, but occasionally they break or leak. Unprotected vaginal or anal intercourse are by far the most risky sexual activities, but viruses in semen can get into the bloodstream through a sore on your hand or a cut in your mouth as you caress your partner to orgasm. You might believe you are in a monogamous relationship, but your partner of thirty years could be having a secret affair. *Safer sex* is sexual activity that does not include exposure to a partner's body fluids. A penis should not enter a vagina or an anus without being fully sheathed by a condom. It is not safe to have penetration for a few minutes, pull out, and then put on a condom before ejaculation.

Although oral sex is less risky for some STDs than vaginal or anal sex, germs from semen or vaginal fluid that contact the mucous membranes of the mouth can enter a partner's bloodstream and cause an infection. A *latex* condom—not the variety made out of natural materials—should be worn over the penis during oral sex. Mint-flavored condoms are now available so that the rubber taste is less of a problem. Dental dams are squares of thin latex that can be stretched across a woman's vulva for safer oral sex. Again, some are flavored, and catalogs even sell a garter belt to hold the latex in place! Try a condom store or sex toy catalog (see Resources under Products to Enhance Sex).

To maximize safety, you can wear thin latex gloves when you caress your partner's genital area. Then a virus such as HIV cannot enter your bloodstream through a cut in your skin. Latex condoms or gloves need lubrication. It is crucial that the lubricant be *water-based* because oil or petroleum jelly can damage latex products. Partners who share vibrators or other sex toys should, before sharing, clean them thoroughly with a detergent that contains nonoxynol-9 (a chemical that can combat viruses including HIV) and should also cover them with condoms for each use.

Although viruses and bacteria are present in saliva, deep kissing mouth to mouth is regarded as low on the scale of risk of transmitting STDs. It is one of those activities that is safer but cannot be declared 100 percent safe.

Having safer sex might seem like such a hassle that you wonder if it is worth having sex at all. Even highly aware men in the gay community sometimes risk their lives by having unprotected sex with partners who could be HIV positive. People who typically use alcohol or street drugs in sexual situations are less likely to have the presence of mind to protect themselves.

Single people worry that a new partner will be turned off by a request to have safer sex. It is difficult enough to discuss your cancer history with a potential mate, let alone ask him or her about STDs and condoms. If your mate has been abusive in the past, you might rightfully fear violence or, at least, verbal abuse when you ask to use a condom.

Because safer sex is so important, I recommend you take a look at some of the books and videos that are available (see Resources) to teach skills on asking assertively for safer sex and to suggest lovemaking techniques that make safer sex more erotic and pleasurable.

Joellen knew she was not the only 19-year-old with cancer, but, around her college campus, that was how she felt. She was having chemotherapy for Hodgkin's disease. Classmates who did not know her story often assumed she had shaved her head for the sake of fashion. With her baldness and several earrings in each earlobe, Joellen was a striking young woman.

She met Reid in the campus co-op grocery store, over the eggplants. It took about three evenings together before Joellen told Reid about her cancer. She waited several more weeks to make sure he was really interested in a relationship before getting sexually involved.

Joellen always intended to ask Reid to use condoms, but she was a little taken aback that he brought it up first, when they only had their shirts off. "You aren't like . . . scared you could get cancer from me, are you?" she asked worriedly. Reid reassured her that he was only worried about preventing pregnancy. Joellen thanked him for his thoughtfulness. In fact, she had stashed condoms right in her bedside table, and the couple soon found that condoms were no barrier to enjoying each other.

Part I of this book has reviewed what you need to know about being sexually active after cancer. Many people develop a sexual problem related to their cancer treatment, however. Part II will explain the causes of the most common sexual difficulties and will suggest ways to overcome them.

PART II

IS THERE A PROBLEM? WHY IT HAPPENED AND HOW TO FIX IT

7

Getting the Help You Need for a Sexual Problem

Perhaps you tried the suggestions in Part I on talking about sex with your partner and on getting back to an active sex life, but you found that something was still not right. Part II gives you information on and suggests solutions for the most common sexual problems after cancer treatment: loss of desire for sex, erection problems, trouble with orgasm, and pain during sex. This chapter suggests general strategies for finding help for a sexual problem. No matter what the sexual difficulty is, you will have to decide whether to try a self-help approach or to explore getting treatment from a health professional.

Self-Help

You can often resolve your own sexual problems. The ingredients of self-help include:

- Getting accurate information
- Trying one or more specific remedies until you find one that works for you
- Getting cooperation from a caring partner

Some of the remedies suggested here just involve working on your own thoughts or feelings. Others are designed for partners to try out. If you do not have a sexual partner, you might want to read Chapter 28 on single people after cancer.

Professional Help

You need professional help in order to get medical treatment for a sexual problem. You might also need professional help if you tried the suggestions in this book but remain unsatisfied with your sex life. It is very hard to find a specialist expert in both sexual problems and in cancer. In fact, if you read this book carefully, you might end up educating your specialist at times. You might even want to show parts of this book to professionals who are treating you.

Your Primary Doctor

With the increasing role of managed care in health settings, you might need to consult your primary care provider about a sexual problem. This physician could be your family doctor or, in some cases, the oncology specialist who manages your cancer treatment. Some general practitioners or oncologists are very sensitive and knowledgeable about sexual issues, but others dislike even discussing the topic. If your primary care physician cannot answer your questions, ask for a referral to a specialist. Sometimes, you might be faced with paying for the specialist out of your pocket if your insurance will not cover the services you need.

Medical Specialists

Specific sexual problems can be evaluated and treated by a medical specialist.

- *Urologists* are the medical specialists most likely to evaluate and treat loss of desire and erection problems in men.
- *Gynecologists* assess women's problems with desire or pain with intercourse.
- Your oncology specialist might be able to help with a sexual problem related directly to your cancer treatment.

Even specialists vary greatly in their expertise about sexual problems. How can you find a specialist who is knowledgeable? Try asking your family doctor about specialists in your community. Call your county or state medical society—some have referral services that can help you match your problem to a physician's area of interest. Some cancer centers have medical specialists who treat sexual problems after cancer. If there is a medical school nearby, call its relevant department and ask if anyone on the faculty has the expertise you need.

Mental Health Specialists

Mental health professionals trained in sex therapy can help you improve your sexual communication, adjust to changes in your sex life after cancer treatment, or resolve sexual problems that are related to anxiety. Sex therapy is a short-term, action-oriented form of psychotherapy. Typically a couple comes for an hour-long session once a week or once every two weeks for five to twenty sessions. The therapist gives assignments to do at home, for example, reading books about sexuality, trying touching exercises that are designed to take away the pressure to perform during sex, or practicing better sexual communication skills. (See Chapter 5 for some of the sensate focus exercises that form the cornerstone of sex therapy.)

You can check to see if the hospital or cancer center where you received your treatment has a mental health professional on staff who provides help with sexual problems. You can get lists of mental health professionals in your area with training in sex therapy from several professional organizations (see Resources under Information Networks). It can be difficult to find a well-trained sex therapy specialist outside of urban areas, however. Remember that basic mental health training, such as a master's degree in social work (M.S.W.), board certification in psychiatry, or a doctorate degree in psychology (Ph.D. or Psy.D.), along with state psychologist licensing are important qualifications for anyone who is providing sexual counseling. Mental health professionals who treat sexual problems never have sexual contact with their patients. Sex between therapist and patient violates legal and ethical standards.

Insurance coverage for mental health services often involves a higher co-payment than for other medical care. Some policies also refuse to pay for sex therapy or for any treatment of sexual dysfunctions. To avoid an unpleasant surprise when you get your bill, check the fine print of your mental health insurance exclusions before you make an appointment.

The ideas in this chapter on getting help for a sexual problem can apply to any of the difficulties discussed in this part of the book. The next few chapters will help you understand how cancer treatment causes sexual problems and will provide information on the types of solutions available.

8

Where Did My Libido Go?

Loss of desire for sex is one of the most common sexual problems after cancer treatment. It is a complex problem that often has multiple causes. In Chapter 1, we discussed how emotional factors contribute to sexual desire problems. Here we focus on the ways that cancer treatment interferes medically with sexual desire.

Feeling Lousy

It is hard to get in the mood for sex when you are generally feeling lousy. Any cancer treatment that produces fatigue, chronic pain, nausea, or weakness can decrease your interest in sex. Common examples include treatments with combination chemotherapy, biological response modifiers (such as interleukin-2 or alpha-interferon), or bone marrow transplant. Remember that the tougher and more prolonged the therapy, the longer it takes to recover a feeling of physical health and well-being. Sexual desire often returns as you regain a more normal level of energy.

The Brain and Sexual Desire

Knowledge about how the brain controls sexuality is limited. Loss of interest in sex is a common problem after surgery, radiation therapy, or chemotherapy for brain tumors, but it is difficult to predict the impact of treatment for any particular person.

Medications That Decrease Desire

Prescription medications can reduce your desire for sex. Sometimes you can change to a different type or dose of medication or stop taking it altogether. Often the intended benefits of the drug outweigh its annoying side effects, however. If you suspect one of your medications is interfering with your sex life, the first thing to do is to discuss your concern with the physician who prescribed it. It is never a good idea to reduce your dose of a medicine or to stop taking it without getting the advice of your doctor.

Narcotics

When given in large doses, narcotic pain medications can decrease sexual desire. These prescription pain relievers are related either to natural morphine or to man-made compounds that act in the body like morphine. Men or women who need narcotics for pain relief are not addicted to their medications. When cancer is advanced, however, people often develop a tolerance to narcotic pain relievers and need an increasingly higher dose to be free of discomfort. For those who still want to stay sexually active, the sexual side effects of the pain medication are annoying but inescapable. Some of the more commonly prescribed narcotic pain medications include Demerol (meperidine hydrochloride), Darvocet (propoxyphene napsylate), Dilaudid (hydromorphone hydrochloride), or Percocet (oxycodone and acetaminophen).

Six years after Laurel's breast cancer was first diagnosed, she developed severe back pain. A bone scan showed that her breast cancer had spread to the bones of her spine. She had two types of chemotherapy and also took tamoxifen, but the cancer continued to advance. Laurel knew she was just buying time but wanted to live as long as she could continue to enjoy her life. Because she was often in pain, Laurel's oncologist prescribed narcotic medication. He told her not to worry about becoming dependent on it, but to use as much as she needed to stay comfortable.

Laurel and her husband, Gary, had stayed sexually active over the years since her cancer, and made love at least once every couple of weeks. Although Laurel often felt drowsy, she found that she could still enjoy sex if she timed lovemaking to begin a few minutes after she took her medication. Then she was almost free of pain but still alert enough so that she did not fall asleep during foreplay. Although Laurel did not feel much drive to have intercourse or orgasms, it was very important to her to give pleasure to Gary. She also felt a strong need to feel Gary's arms around her and to lie curved against his body. Knowing that their remaining time together was limited made each sensation precious.

Drugs for Nausea

Although nausea itself certainly can ruin a sexy mood, some of the medications used to prevent or relieve it also interfere with sexual desire. Some medications have sexual side effects mainly because they are tranquilizing. Compazine (prochlorperazine) and another common antinausea drug, Reglan (metoclopramide), also might temporarily increase levels of the hormone prolactin. Prolactin is made in the *pituitary gland* (a small structure under the base of the brain; in women, prolactin helps with milk production). In men and women, high prolactin levels appear to limit desire for sex. If a kidney function is poor after cancer treatment, prolactin levels also might be higher than normal. A blood test can measure prolactin.

Newer antinausea drugs, Zofran (ondansetron hydrochloride) and Kytril (granisetron hydrochloride), have a different action on brain chemicals. Their impact on sexuality is not yet known. Tagamet (cimetidine) is used to prevent or treat stomach ulcers or heartburn. It interferes with testosterone and, in high doses, can depress sexual desire.

Tranquilizers and Antidepressants

Tranquilizers and antidepressants can help cancer patients with sleep, mood, anxiety, or chronic pain. These medications act in the brain to change levels of *neurotransmitters*, chemicals that carry messages from one brain cell to another.

Most drugs used to treat anxiety, such as Ativan (lorazepam), Buspar (buspirone hydrochloride), Klonopin (clonazepam), Valium (diazepam), or Xanax (alprazolam), also decrease sexual desire in men and women.

Antidepressants can have a variety of sexual side effects. On one hand, if depression was decreasing sexual desire, then taking an antidepressant might actually help sexual feelings to return. On the other hand, antidepressants can interfere with desire for sex, especially some of the newer ones that increase the levels of the neurotransmitter serotonin. These medications, called *selective serotonin reuptake inhibitors* (SSRIs), include Paxil (paroxetine hydrochloride), Prozac (fluoxetine hydrochloride), or Zoloft (sertraline hydrochloride).

Blood Pressure Medicines

Although heart disease and hypertension are rarely directly linked to cancer, they are common illnesses among older men and women. *Beta-blockers*, medications that reduce blood pressure and are often used for heart disease, cause fatigue and reduce sexual desire. Beta-blockers include Inderal (propranolol hydrochloride), Corgard (nadolol), Lopressor (metoprolol tartrate), Tenormin (atenolol), and Visken (pindolol).

Upsetting the Hormonal Balance in Men

The most common physical way that cancer treatments decrease sexual desire is by influencing the balance of sex hormones. Remember from Chapter 2 that men need a minimum amount of testosterone to have normal sexual desire, erections, and sexual sensation. Luckily, the Leydig cells in the testicles that produce testosterone are not easily damaged by chemotherapy or radiation. A few men do end up with abnormally low hormone levels, however. Typical symptoms would include loss of desire for sex, trouble getting erections or reaching orgasm, hot flashes, irritability, and reduced beard growth.

Testicular Cancer

Men with testicular cancer typically have a tumor in only one testicle, which is then removed surgically. The remaining testicle usually can produce enough testosterone to make up for losing the other. Occasionally, however, a man loses both testicles to cancer or is left with one testicle that had never functioned very well. Then his testosterone levels may be abnormally low.

Bone Marrow Transplant

Whole body irradiation or very strong chemotherapy given before a bone marrow transplant can sometimes decrease testosterone production. After a bone marrow transplant from a donor, graft versus host disease can also disrupt hormones. For some men, the damage is temporary, and hormone levels recover. For other men, the hormone loss might be permanent.

Radiation to the Pelvis

Men who have radiation therapy to the pelvis for cancer of the prostate, colon, or bladder might have a temporary decrease in testosterone because of radiation scatter to the testicles. The testicles are not the direct target of radiation and are protected with lead shields during the treatment. However, radiation bounces off internal organs very much like a bullet ricochets when it hits a wall. The testicles still end up getting a small dose. Most men recover normal levels of testosterone within six months of the end of radiation therapy to the pelvis. Radiation directly to a testicle (sometimes used for seminoma or childhood leukemia) can do more permanent damage.

Hormone Therapy for Prostate Cancer

Because prostate cancer is sensitive to testosterone (in other words, most prostate cancer cells require testosterone in their diet), it can be treated by eliminating as much testosterone as possible in the bloodstream. Some men have both testicles removed surgically, whereas others take shots of a substance called a *luteinizing hormone releasing hormone* (LHRH) agonist, such as Lupron or Goserelin, that shuts down the testicles' testosterone factory. In the past, the female hormone estrogen was also commonly prescribed, but it is used more rarely now because it increases the risk of heart disease and stroke. Some men are also given drugs like Flutamide or Casodex that block the action of testosterone at the level of the cell. These drugs are often combined with LHRH agonists.

All of these hormone therapies have a similar impact on men's sex lives. About 80 percent of men give up on sexual activity and say that they feel little or no desire for sex. The remaining 20 percent of men manage to stay sexually active. They often say that it takes stronger stimulation to get in the mood for sex, for example, watching an erotic video, having a good deal of foreplay, or reading stories that promote sexual fantasies. They might take longer to get an erection than in the past, or their erections might be less firm. Most of these men can reach an orgasm, but it takes more time and effort than before. Typically, they ejaculate little or no semen.

Most men on hormone therapy are elderly, but, in my experience, it is often those under age 65 who manage to enjoy sex despite treatment. Perhaps they start out with more frequent sexual desire, so that the loss of testosterone still leaves them a reserve of interest in their mental "sex account."

Premature Menopause and Sexual Desire

Damage to the ovaries from radiation therapy to the pelvis or from chemotherapy can bring on premature menopause (discussed in detail in Chapter 19). Some women also have both ovaries removed surgically as part of their cancer treatment. Without the androgen hormones made by the ovaries, women might notice a loss of sexual desire, although the androgen hormones made by the adrenal glands also help to maintain sexual desire. If a woman takes steroids such as prednisone as part of her chemotherapy, androgen production by the adrenal glands can be temporarily interrupted as well.

The late Dr. Helen Singer Kaplan, a well-known psychiatrist and sex therapist in New York, described a group of women who came to her complaining of low sexual desire after cancer chemotherapy. Blood tests showed that some of these women had little or no testosterone. Dr. Kaplan found that injections of a small amount of testosterone every two weeks often restored these women's sexual desire.

Amy thought several times that she would not survive her bone marrow transplant for acute myelogenous leukemia (AML). On some days, she felt so dreadful, between terrible irritation of her mouth and throat and shaking chills from the antifungal drugs she was given, that she almost wished she would not survive. After six weeks in the hospital, however, Amy came home. Her ordeal was not yet over, however. To treat graft versus host disease, she had to take steroids that gave her severe acne and cheeks like a chipmunk. Her eyes and mouth were chronically dry, and she felt weak and nauseated. Diarrhea was also a problem. Needless to say, sex was not high on her list of priorities, even though she and her husband had only been married for five years.

By the time she had been home for six months, Amy was beginning to feel that she might be healthy again someday. She and her husband began cuddling more and tried some sexual touching. Amy still felt little interest in sex, however. A blood test showed only low levels of testosterone, but she was reluctant to try taking hormones when she was still on so many medications, including an antidepressant and drugs to relieve nausea. After several more months, Amy felt some return of sexual desire and was able to reach orgasm again. Amy's capacity to enjoy sex improved very slowly along with her general health. There were so many factors interfering with her desire that no pill or shot could act as a magic potion to restore it. Love, patience, and good sexual communication were more important than hormones.

9

Enhancing Sexual Desire after Cancer

Because loss of sexual desire after cancer often results from more than one cause, restoring libido typically takes more than one, simple treatment. In this chapter, I suggest a variety of ways to stimulate sexual desire or to get more pleasure out of sex.

Pills and Potions

Have you ever asked your doctor to prescribe a pill to boost your sexual desire? The media regularly present stories about sensational, sex-enhancing drugs. Unfortunately, there is no magic pill. If one existed, the pharmaceutical company that owned the patent would zoom to the top of the stock market. You can imagine the research dollars invested in searching for a true *aphrodisiac* (a substance that would increase men's or women's interest in sex).

If you have lost your desire for sex as part of a more general depression, antidepressant medication will sometimes improve your desire along with your mood. Unfortunately, many antidepressants also can blunt sexual desire, interfere with erections in men, or make it difficult for men or women to reach an orgasm. If one antidepressant interferes with sex, you could try an alternative one. Wellbutrin (buproprion) and Desyrel (trazodone) are two that seem to have fewer sexual side effects.

A prescription medication containing yohimbine (Yocon), a chemical found in the bark of an African tree, is often mentioned as an aphrodisiac. Scientific research has only suggested a weak effect of yohimbine on human sexual responsiveness, however. Rather than increasing sexual desire, yohimbine simply appears to make it somewhat easier for men to get erections in a minority of cases—and typically only if the erection problem is based on anxiety. Some psychiatrists have found that adding yohimbine to antidepressant therapy can relieve some of the negative sexual side effects.

Other herbs or chemicals advertised in health food stores as sexual stimulants have not been scientifically proven to be effective. Taking vitamins or zinc will not improve your sex life and can be harmful to your health if you exceed the maximum recommended dose.

Do You Need Extra Testosterone?

Replacement androgen hormones might help sexual desire in a small minority of men or women, but only if baseline hormone levels are abnormally low. Most men and women retain normal testosterone levels after cancer treatment. If you have noticed a general loss of sexual interest, a simple blood test can measure total serum testosterone (the general amount in your bloodstream) and free testosterone (the amount that is biologically active and, thus, able to enter target cells in your brain to promote sexual desire).

Testosterone for Men

Testosterone replacement for men is quite routine. Testosterone is usually given in an injection once or twice a month or through a special patch that glues on to the skin of the scrotum or the abdomen. A man has to shave the area where he places the patch, and the treatment is more expensive, but many men like avoiding shots. Testosterone given in pill form does not get absorbed as well by the body and can sometimes damage a man's liver.

Although men sometimes take testosterone when their own levels are just on the low side, it is not a good idea. Not only does extra testosterone rarely help a man's sex life, but it can be hazardous to his health. The steroids that body builders take illegally are types of testosterone. In large doses, they actually shut down a man's interest in sex and cause his testicles to shrink in size. If a man has a prostate cancer that has not been diagnosed, taking extra testosterone could also stimulate the cancer cells to grow and spread. After prostate cancer is treated, men should not take replacement testosterone because of the concern that it could reactivate any remaining cancer cells.

Testosterone for Women

Because women produce only low levels of androgens, there is confusion about how much they need to maintain normal sexual desire. Some women use a low dose of injectable hormone. There is no testosterone patch on the market with a dose that is right for women. As in men, the pill form of testosterone might be less safe and effective than the injectable type, but it is still commonly prescribed. At high doses, testosterone can have masculinizing side effects in women, such as increased growth of facial hair, thinning of scalp hair, enlargement of the clitoris, deepening of the voice, and acne. In the small doses of testosterone used for hormone replacement, these side effects would be quite unusual; but it is common for women to notice oilier skin and to have less favorable cholesterol ratios.

The safety of testosterone replacement for women after breast cancer has not been tested, and testosterone replacement could be more risky than estrogen replacement. Although high doses of testosterone have been used to treat advanced breast cancer, other research suggests that testosterone might increase women's breast cancer risk. Women who have their ovaries destroyed by radiation therapy for cancer in the pelvic area have a lower chance of developing breast cancer later in their lives. One explanation is that the lack of androgens from the ovaries reduces breast cancer risk. Another line of research suggests that women who develop breast cancer have unusually high androgen levels in their bloodstream.

Is It Working?

If you are using replacement testosterone, its sexual stimulant effect should be obvious within the first two or three days. If you do not feel anything by that time, it is probably not going to have a positive impact on your sexual desire. Typically, sexual desire wanes again as your dose of testosterone wears off. It can be tricky to find the right dose of hormone. People on injections often notice a peak of desire soon after the shot and a valley before the next one is due. For men, the patch might provide a more even level of libido.

Promoting Desire in Your Daily Routine

Because few men or women achieve better sex through chemistry, it is important to use some psychology to promote sexual desire after cancer treatment. One factor that often interferes with desire is feeling like a medical patient instead of a vital, sexy person. During cancer treatment, most people endure physical pain and many indignities involving loss of control over daily life. Feeling sexual again is easier if you can experience pleasure from your body. If your desire for sex is low, here are some strategies to get into the mood.

Work Out!

Sexual desire is stronger when you are in good physical condition. Perhaps there are limits to how much you can exercise or improve your health, but consider what your options are. Can you dance, walk, or swim regularly? Even if you have very limited stamina, a physical therapist might be able to suggest exercises to keep up some flexibility and strength. Increasingly, physical therapy is a part of rehabilitation for cancer patients. If you have given up a sport you enjoyed, are you ready to return to it? If you are a golfer, perhaps you need to use a cart or a caddie or to play nine holes instead of eighteen. If you were a jogger, maybe you need to start out with walking instead.

Janine attended aerobics classes four times a week until her symptoms of ovarian cancer slowed her down. At forty-five, she was proud of her tight body and young appearance and totally unprepared for the way cancer treatment took over her life. After major pelvic surgery, she underwent months of chemotherapy. Even the newer antinausea drugs could not keep her from feeling sick. She quit her job as a freelance illustrator for children's books. Between eating bland snacks to combat nausea and lack of activity, she gained fifteen pounds. Friends offered to help her shop for wigs or scarves, but Janine was so depressed that she hardly left the house, except to go to the hospital for her treatments. She was sure she was dying.

After her second-look surgery found no remaining cancer, Janine was told she was finished with cancer treatment. Her hair started to grow back and she no longer felt sick all the time, but she was still depressed. Her husband and sister gave Janine a health club membership to celebrate her recovery. Janine tried the aerobics class once. She hated the way she looked in her exercise clothes and felt frustrated that she had such poor stamina. Instead of taking a place in the front row as had been her habit in the past, she put her mat in the back corner near the door.

Janine's neighbor Ruth had an inspiration. Instead of pushing Janine to get out more, Ruth asked Janine for help. "I've gained ten pounds this winter," Ruth said, "and I'm having a terrible time motivating myself to exercise. Would you be willing to take a walk with me every day?" Ruth was considerably heavier than Janine and far less athletic. Janine agreed readily to help her friend, and the two began to walk daily. As Ruth had hoped, their walks helped Janine get interested in more vigorous exercise. Janine started dressing and taking care of herself like she had before her cancer. And Ruth also ended up losing the weight she had recently put on!

Don't Take Your Body for Granted

Few Americans, especially women, feel satisfied with their appearance. The media hold up a standard of beauty and fitness hardly anyone can match. People typically rate their own physical attractiveness several points lower than the judgments of outside observers. Even the young and healthy criticize themselves harshly. How much more difficult it becomes to love and enjoy one's body after an illness. The more negatively you feel about your body, the more difficult it becomes to feel sexual. Thoughts about extra weight, wrinkles, scars, or other changes can distract you in the middle of lovemaking.

A different way to think about your body is to rejoice in all the ways that it remains healthy and whole. Perhaps you have lost a testicle, but you still can hit a home run. You might have a colostomy, but you also have terrific legs. Your hair has fallen out, but your lymph nodes have returned to normal size. What can you do to celebrate your body? How can you be extra nice to the only body you will ever have? Having a brush with death can make the pleasures of living more vivid and intense.

Delight Your Senses

Sexual pleasure depends in part on giving yourself permission to enjoy your senses. Think of each sense and the pleasure it can give you. For visual enjoyment, take extra time to dress in a favorite outfit and notice how nice you look. Ask your partner to wear something special that puts you in the mood for sex. To delight your sense of smell, take a bubble bath or splash on some cologne. Rub scented body lotion on your partner before bedtime. To revel in touch, ask your partner to stroke your hair or your back. Run your hands over your partner's body and notice the smooth shapes or soft skin. For the pleasure of sound, put on your favorite music next time you make love. Ask your partner to whisper something sexy in your ear. To include taste, kiss your partner in several places and notice how each one tastes. Eat a favorite food with your partner in bed.

> Bonnie was still in the middle of chemotherapy for lymphoma. One weekend between courses of treatment, her mother offered to take the children overnight to give Bonnie and her husband, Jeff, some private time. The couple ordered pizza delivered so that neither would have to spend energy cooking. After dinner they watched a romantic comedy on video and then went up to their bedroom. Bonnie had prepared the tape player with a favorite rock album from their dating years. Bonnie was not very happy with the way she looked because of hair loss and having a catheter in her shoulder. She put a scented candle in the bedroom so that she would feel less self-conscious and also decided to wear a silk kimono and let Jeff caress her underneath it. Bonnie usually avoided alcohol because it made her drowsy on top of her medication, but she sipped a little champagne, just for the taste and to feel she and Jeff were celebrating. The couple spent a long time just kissing and stroking each other's bodies before they finally had intercourse. Afterward, Bonnie was surprised at how much she had enjoyed the evening.

Slow-Cook Your Desire

In the busy lives of most couples, thoughts about sex quickly get dismissed, and lovemaking becomes a quickie after the eleven o'clock news. A recent survey of adults aged 18 to 59 in the United States found that only a third have sex once a week or more. Sex therapists often suggest that sexual desire needs to simmer on the back burner for a while so that it takes less effort to turn up the flame when the time is right. What can you do to keep your home fires burning?

Tune in to the sexual signals that surround you. For some, the sexual images in advertisements and in the media are turn-ons, but for others they are turn-offs. Perhaps reading a novel or seeing a movie with a good love scene is more arousing for you. Some people prefer subtle doses of sex, while others like the most explicit erotica. If there is a story, picture, or film that aroused you in the past, take some time to enjoy it on a day when you hope to try sex with your partner.

Do you have a personal sexual fantasy? Having an erotic image in your mind can help to distract you from anxiety or pain as you get ready for sex. The more vivid your fantasy, the more arousing it can be. If you feel guilty about fantasizing, perhaps you can focus on a good memory of sex with your current partner, or you can imagine the two of you in an especially romantic setting. In your fantasy, you can be just as you are, an improved version of yourself, or someone else entirely! If you have trouble developing a sexual fantasy, you might want to read through collections of short erotic stories or sexual fantasies. A good mail order source of erotic books or videos is The Sexuality Library (see Resources under Products to Enhance Sex).

Think about activities that put you in the mood for sex. Perhaps the physical glow you get from dancing or playing tennis can spill over into feeling sexual desire. Maybe you need some private time just to relax so that you can turn your attention later to your partner. If your energy is limited, scheduling time to lie down or nap before trying sex might help. If you have sore joints or back pain, a bath or massage can be a helpful prelude to lovemaking.

Val's favorite activity in the world was to go see a professional ice hockey game in the winter. He and his brothers had season tickets. The wives stayed home while the men shouted themselves hoarse, but Val's wife, Paula, could always count on his waking her up for a great session of sex when he came home. Even though he tasted like hot dogs and beer, these were some of their best lovemaking times. Paula joked that Val must have some Roman ancestors because bloody brawls seemed to really turn him on.

Val was diagnosed with acute leukemia and went through a bone marrow transplant complicated by a near-fatal episode of pneumonia. Even when he came home after almost three months in the hospital, it took another few weeks before he was back at work part-time or had the stamina for any leisure fun. Val and Paula had tried some sexual activity once or twice, but Val had trouble getting an erection. He did not initiate sex, and Paula did not want to pressure him. Then hockey season started. The night of the first game, Val's brothers came to pick him up. Paula did not want to get her hopes up or make Paul think she expected him to perform for her sexually, so she arranged to go to a concert with one of her woman friends. When she arrived home, Val was already in bed. Paula tiptoed into the bedroom and slipped under the covers. She was surprised and delighted when Val put his arms around her and gave her a kiss that tasted of mustard, sausage, and ale.

What can you do to feel your most attractive? If you want to get in the mood for sex, is there something you can wear that helps you feel more sexual? If you have scars or physical changes from your cancer treatment, do you prefer to camouflage them or to learn to feel positive about them as badges of your survival? Do you enjoy wearing perfume or aftershave? What about sexy lingerie if you are a woman or silk boxer shorts, bikini briefs, or a special bathrobe if you are a man?

You can also turn up the heat on your desire by taking brief "making out" breaks with your partner or by caressing your own body in private (to warm up your desire for partner sex, stop short of orgasm).

Making Sex More Erotic

If you begin sex without having a strong amount of desire, you might find it effortful to get fully aroused or to reach orgasm. This type of problem is quite common in men or women after cancer treatment. In recent years, magazine articles and talk shows have touted variety in sex, giving the message that routine sex is a warning sign of impending divorce and premature aging. The reality, however, is that most people have sex lives that are not very frequent or varied. Couples include the same types of kissing and caressing in the same order during their foreplay, have intercourse in one or two positions each time, and even have sex at one typical time of day or on one day of the week. Most married couples are happy with this pattern, but it can become a problem if cancer leaves you with a sexual response that is weak or sluggish.

Perhaps some extra mental or physical sexual stimulation would help you to get a better erection or to lubricate more or would help make it easier to reach an orgasm. In Chapter 5, we suggested spending a longer time on foreplay, giving each other more feedback on the types of hand caressing or oral stimulation that feels best, or varying positions for intercourse. You also might find inspiration by browsing in a store or catalog that sells sex toys, such as vibrators, lingerie, videos, lubricants, and fancy condoms. Such items used to be marketed only in adult bookstores in sleazy neighborhoods that most people felt embarrassed or unsafe to visit. Now stores that sell sexy lingerie or other sexual aids are often found in suburban shopping malls. A number of mail order catalogs are also available, including some that market videotapes providing education on sexual techniques or suggestions for overcoming sexual problems (see Resources under Products to Enhance Sex).

Sometimes the desire for sex remains strong, but cancer treatment interferes with some aspect of sexual performance or pleasure. The next two chapters discuss causes and treatment of erection problems, men's most dreaded sexual difficulty.

10

Causes of Erection Problems

The most common sexual problem after cancer treatment in men is difficulty getting or keeping erections. Most of these problems have a medical basis; that is, cancer treatment has permanently damaged the hormones, nerves, or blood vessels involved in erection. Older men also might have erection problems due to medical causes unrelated to their cancer treatment. At age 40, only about 20 percent of American men have a significant erection problem; but by age 70, half of men do. Sometimes, erection problems after cancer are only temporary, or they can actually be caused by psychological factors. Erection problems can result in great emotional pain for men. They not only interfere with sexual pleasure, but also can damage self-esteem.

Cancer Treatment and Performance Anxiety

Cancer treatment can cause performance anxiety for a man. Perhaps he fears being unable to function the first time he has sex after cancer. If he does run into a problem, he might start to worry about what will happen the next time he tries sex. Instead of enjoying his erotic sensations, he starts to become a "penis watcher"—Is it getting hard? Am I ready to start intercourse? Will it stay up? Foreplay becomes a frantic effort to get an erection, and he tries penetration the minute he thinks he can manage it.

One hallmark of performance anxiety is having distracting thoughts about your erection when you are trying to enjoy sex. Another important feature is feeling ashamed of your failure to perform. You can develop performance anxiety even if a medical problem is interfering with erections. Here are some signs that your problem might be based on anxiety:

- You wake up in the middle of the night or in the morning with a firm erection.
- You get an erection without effort in a situation when you do not expect to have sex.
- Your erections are pretty normal if you touch yourself in private or watch an erotic videotape, but they are poor when you are with a partner.
- Your erections are firm with one partner but are abnormal with a different one.
- You have not had a cancer treatment known to damage erection capacity.

Low Testosterone and Erection Problems

If a man's hormone levels are abnormal, his ability to get and keep good erections is often affected. Typically he will notice a loss of desire for sex, will have few or no erections on waking from sleep, and will find it quite a chore to get and keep an erection. As was discussed in Chapter 8, most men continue to have normal levels of testosterone or prolactin, despite cancer treatment or aging. Men on hormone therapy for prostate cancer are, of course, an exception. Diagnosing and correcting hormone abnormalities can improve erections.

Medications That Interfere with Erections

A number of medications are known to cause problems with erections. For men after cancer, common ones include the following:

Tranquilizers

Your family doctor or oncologist might prescribe medication to promote sleep or decrease nervousness. These tranquilizers can interfere with erections indirectly, by causing drowsiness and lack of desire for sex, or directly, by interfering with the nervous system impulses that control erection.

Antidepressants

Most antidepressants can interfere with erections for a minority of men. Erection problems are less common with a newer class of antidepressants, the serotonin reuptake inhibitors, including Prozac, Paxil, and Zoloft, but loss of desire for sex and problems reaching orgasm are quite common. Two other antidepressants, Wellbutrin and Desyrel, seem to have fewer sexual side effects than many others. Their effectiveness in treating depression might not always be optimal, however. Wellbutrin can occasionally cause seizures. Some men who take Desyrel have had a problem called *priapism*, an erection that will not go down. Although priapism might sound like a bonus rather than a drawback, in fact, it becomes a medical emergency and can result in permanent scarring of the penis.

Medication for Delirium

Sometimes a cancer treatment causes temporary mental confusion called *delirium*. Symptoms can include delusions, hallucinations, and problems with memory. Older people who have surgery or endure long hospitalizations are especially vulnerable. The most common medication prescribed in this situation is Haldol (haloperidol), a powerful drug also used to treat psychiatric disorders such as schizophrenia. Haldol might be continued for a while, even when the confusion is clearing up. Haldol can interfere with sexual desire and might cause erection problems or trouble with ejaculation in men. These side effects should disappear after the medication is discontinued.

Antibiotics

Although cancer patients often take powerful antibiotics, they rarely have any impact on sexual function. One exception is the drug Nizoral (ketoconazole), used to combat fungal infections. Nizoral suppresses testosterone production and, therefore, can interfere with sexual desire and other aspects of sexual function. Hormone levels recover when Nizoral is no longer needed.

Drugs to Treat High Blood Pressure and Heart Disease

Heart disease and hypertension are rarely directly linked to cancer but are common illnesses among older men. Many medications used to lower blood pressure are notorious in causing erection problems. Sexual side effects are fairly common when men are given beta-blockers (e.g., Inderal or Lopressor) or blood pressure medications based on methyldopa (Aldomet and Aldoclor), reserpine (Hydropres and Regroton), clonidine (Catapres), or guanethidine (Esimil and Ismelin).

Calcium channel blockers are less likely to cause sexual problems and include Calan, Cardizem, and Procardia. Lower rates of sexual side effects are also seen with the angiotensin converting enzyme inhibitors (often abbreviated as ACE inhibitors). These medications include Accupril, Capoten, Monopril, and Vasotec.

Diuretics are drugs that increase the production of urine. They are given to lower blood pressure or sometimes to decrease water retention related to heart failure or other medical illnesses. Most diuretics appear to interfere with erections in some of the men who take them.

Damage from Pelvic Cancer Surgery

It was only in the early 1980s that two urologist researchers, Tom Lue, M.D., of the University of California at San Francisco, and Patrick Walsh, M.D., of Johns Hopkins University Medical School, traced the nerve pathways involved in erection and discovered exactly why most men lost the ability to have firm erections after radical cancer surgery in the pelvis. Operations that might involve cutting through important bundles of nerves on the left and right sides of the rear of the prostate include the following:

- Radical prostatectomy—removing the prostate and seminal vesicles for prostate cancer
- Radical cystectomy—removing the bladder, prostate, seminal vesicles, and part or all of the urethra for bladder cancer
- Abdominoperineal resection—removing the colon and part or all of the rectum for colorectal cancer
- Total pelvic exenteration—a rare surgery that includes removal of the prostate, seminal vesicles, bladder, and colon

When nerve fibers are cut, the effect is like fraying telephone wires at one end. The command from the brain to produce an erection gets weakened or interrupted. Many men still get swelling and enlargement of the penis after surgery, but not enough blood flow to produce a really stiff erection.

When men hear that cancer surgery could damage nerves involved in erection, they imagine that the operation will leave them unable to feel desire for sex or to enjoy caressing of the penis. Actually, the nerves that control blood flow to the penis are entirely separate from the sensory nerves responsible for skin sensation, orgasmic pleasure, or ejaculation of semen. Those sensory nerves run along the sides of the pelvis and are not in the central area where the surgeon is working.

After radical cancer surgery, a man's desire for sex should remain normal from a medical point of view. His ability to enjoy touch in the genital area does not decrease. With the right kind of physical and mental stimulation, he should still be able to have all the feeling of orgasm. However, after some of these operations he might have a dry orgasm (see Chapters 2 and 12).

Nerve-Sparing Surgery

Dr. Walsh created a new type of nerve-sparing radical prostate surgery, designed to leave the nerves uncut whenever possible. Nerve-sparing techniques not only increase the percentage of men who recover usable erections, but also decrease bleeding during surgery and result in fewer men who are left with permanent urinary *incontinence* (involuntary loss of control over urination). If a prostate tumor is too close to the crucial area on one side, sometimes at least the nerves can be spared on the other side. Nerve-sparing techniques have now been adopted by many surgeons who perform radical cystectomy or colorectal cancer surgery, but unfortunately total pelvic exenteration is such a big operation that nerve-sparing is not possible.

Will You Recover Erections?

Recovery of erections after nerve-sparing surgery is gradual. Most men need several months to a year, and some have said that improvement continued into the second year after surgery. During this transition period, some men use treatments such as penile injections or vacuum pumps (see Chapter 11) to enhance their erections until nature takes over.

The men most likely to recover good erections are (1) those who had excellent erections before surgery, (2) those who are younger and healthier, and (3) those for whom the surgeon managed to spare the nerves on both the left and right sides. (A more detailed discussion of nerve-sparing radical prostatectomy is found in Chapter 24.)

Damage from Radiation Therapy in the Pelvic Area

Radiation therapy aimed at the pelvic area interferes with erections for a number of men. Most commonly, large doses of pelvic radiation are given to treat prostate cancer, but this therapy is also used at times with cancer of the bladder or colon. Men with the testicular cancer seminoma might get smaller doses of radiation targeted to the scrotum and groin.

When radiation is given from a machine outside the body, it can be aimed very accurately at the tumor, typically using computers to design a target field. Nevertheless, some radiation damage occurs in areas close to the tumor. Radiation causes local irritation as the dose builds up over several weeks of treatments. The healing process then takes months or even years. Tissues that receive a large dose of radiation often develop scarring, called *fibrosis*. Like tough meat, these tissues lose some of their soft and stretchy quality.

When radiation is given to the pelvis, the blood vessels that supply the penis often get a hefty dose. Erection problems may occur if the blood vessels get scarred and narrow, not allowing enough blood to rush into the penis during erection. Scarring inside the cavernous bodies of the penis may also contribute to the problem.

Typically, the sexual changes do not happen overnight or even during the weeks of radiation treatment. Instead, they begin gradually, perhaps six months or a year after the end of radiation therapy as scar tissue develops. The men most likely to develop a severe problem with erection after radiation are the ones who were just barely functioning sexually before their cancer was diagnosed. Their erections might already have been less than firm, and blood flow to the penis might have been marginal. Then the added insult of radiation would make a difficulty into a real problem. Men who are cigarette smokers, who have a history of heart disease or high blood pressure, or who are diabetic are more likely to fall into this high-risk category.

Erection problems are common after radiation therapy for prostate cancer (see Chapter 24 for a detailed discussion). Young men with testicular cancer who have extensive radiation therapy that included the pelvis and upper abdomen are more likely to develop erection problems as they age. Luckily this type of treatment is less common now that chemotherapy for testicular cancer is so effective.

No long-term studies have looked at sexual problems in men who receive high doses of radiation to the whole body for bone marrow transplants or to areas outside the pelvis, for example, for Hodgkin's disease. It is certainly possible that some damage to penile blood flow takes place and may combine with other risk factors to create a higher rate of erection problems when these men reach their middle years.

Damage from Chemotherapy

Chemotherapy drugs rarely play an obvious role in causing erection problems. Certainly some chemotherapy drugs cause nerve damage, but few reports suggest permanent loss of the ability to have erections after their use. As was mentioned earlier, a few men have either temporary or permanent damage to the testicles from chemotherapy and may need some replacement testosterone to function well sexually.

Now that you know how cancer treatment can interfere with erections, we will take a look at the variety of treatments available to restore more normal sexual function to men.

11

How to Mend a Broken Part: Restoring Erections

Great strides have been made in treating erection problems in the past twenty years. None of the current treatments is truly simple, like a pill that will improve erections, but several are quite effective. The bottom line is that almost any man can find a treatment to improve his erections, depending on how much hassle he is willing to endure.

Tests That Can Help You Choose the Right Treatment

As you saw in the preceding chapter, erection problems are to be expected after certain cancer treatments. When the cause of the problem is unclear, however, or if there is a question of which type of treatment will best restore erections, some specialized medical tests can be of help. A urologist who specializes in sexual problems is usually the expert to consult.

Monitoring Erections during Sleep

Normally a man has several firm, lasting erections each night during his sleep. These erections happen during rapid eye movement (REM) sleep, a period in which a man sleeps very deeply and dreams occur. The erections that develop during REM sleep are just a reflex, however, and do not depend on having a dream about sex. Men often awaken in the morning after a period of REM sleep. When they notice their hard erection, they believe it was triggered by a full bladder, but, in fact, the two are just coincidental.

If a man is having erection problems that are caused by anxiety or lack of attraction to a partner, his erections during sleep should remain normal. There are some exceptions to this rule. Men who are severely depressed or who have lost all desire for sex sometimes have poor nighttime erections. If an erection problem has a permanent, medical cause, erections during sleep usually are abnormal. If they occur, they may last a very brief time or not be fully rigid.

Erections during sleep can be monitored using an electronic device called a Rigiscan (Dacomed, Inc.). A man wears a "black box" strapped to his thigh while he sleeps. Two wires each lead to a Velcro loop. One loop is placed around the base of the penis, and the other just under the head of the penis. During the night, the Rigiscan records size changes and rigidity at the base and tip of the penis. When the monitor is plugged into a computer, it prints out a graph of the man's erections across his hours of sleep. Most clinics ask a man to take the Rigiscan home with him and use it for two nights. A familiar setting helps a man sleep more soundly and maximizes the chance of getting good erections.

Rigiscan studies are especially helpful when the recording shows some good, normal erections. A normal study can usually rule out permanent damage to the nerves or blood vessels involved in erection. This kind of result suggests that sex therapy could be helpful in resolving the erection problem. Rigiscan studies can also be used to document that a medically based erection problem exists so that insurance companies will agree to cover treatment for it.

Although home monitoring with a Rigiscan unit is most commonly used, two other types of evaluation are also practiced. A full-scale sleep laboratory evaluation can diagnose sleep problems that may make a home recording inaccurate. At the other end of the spectrum, when a superficial screening of sleep erections is all that is needed, urologists may send a man home with snap gauges (Dacomed, Inc.) for two or three nights. Snap gauges are loops with a Velcro closing and three cellophane snaps in the middle part. If a man gets a firm erection during the night, he will break all three snaps. A weaker erection will only break one or two.

Hormone Tests

The most frequent blood test used to check hormones related to erections is a serum testosterone test. Sometimes a free testosterone value is also ordered to make sure there is enough testosterone in the bloodstream in an active state. Tests for serum prolactin or for thyroid hormones may also be helpful.

Tests of Penile Blood Circulation

Over the past few years, a variety of fancy tests have been invented to measure circulation of blood to the penis. None of these tests is as scientifically accurate as it sounds, and several that were popular in recent years have already fallen out of favor.

The most common test of circulation used these days is the Doppler ultrasound study of the penis. Sound waves are used to create a color picture of blood flow in and out of the penis. Measurements are taken when the penis is not erect and again after an injection of medication to produce erection. The test measures how much arteries expand when blood flow increases during erection. The speed of blood flow into the penis and the amount of outflow during erection are also measured. The Doppler ultrasound may give a better idea of the cause of an erection problem, but results from it rarely change decisions about treatment.

Tests of Nerves Involved in Erection

The nerves that direct blood flow into the penis cannot be tested directly, except during surgery. Despite attempts to invent a test that could diagnose problems in the nervous system involved in erection, none has proven reliable. A brief neurological examination may be helpful to check for symptoms that could indicate a general nervous system problem. Skin sensitivity on the penis can be tested by using a small machine that vibrates gently or produces a weak electrical pulse. This test can be helpful if a man believes his skin sensation has decreased since cancer treatment. For example, some chemotherapy drugs can cause *neuropathy* (nerve damage that results in numbness or tingling in the hands or feet). Occasionally men report that neuropathy symptoms affect their ability to feel pleasure with touch on the penis.

Although cancer treatment that affects the brain or spinal cord may cause changes in sexual function, there is no effective way to measure the impact directly. Doctors can only ask carefully about a man's experiences with sex before his illness and after cancer treatment and then execute a plan based on a commonsense guess about whether he will recover better erections in the future.

Medical Treatments to Restore Erections

The ideal medical treatment would be a pill that would help a man get an erection. In fact, pharmaceutical companies are testing such a pill, but it is not yet on the market. How effective it will be or whether it will work for men whose cancer treatment has damaged nerves or blood vessels involved in erection is not yet known. Perhaps by the time you read this book, we will know more. If an erection-enhancing pill becomes available, you can bet that it will make headlines.

In the meanwhile, there are three medical treatments that are quite effective: vacuum constriction devices, penile injections, and penile prostheses.

Vacuum Constriction Devices

Vacuum constriction devices (VCDs) are most commonly used to treat erection problems that have a medical cause. Because VCDs rarely have long-term side effects, they are sometimes used to treat anxiety-based erection problems also. The hope is that using the VCD will decrease a man's anxiety during sex and allow him to regain better erections in the future. However, it is not known how often men with stress-related erection problems are able to stop using their VCDs or how often they become psychologically dependent on them.

A VCD is a viable option for most men whose cancer treatment has damaged erections. It can be used as soon as a man recovers from radical pelvic surgery. There is no reason to think that using a VCD would delay or prevent recovery of erections after nerve-sparing surgery. A VCD could also be used after radiotherapy to the pelvis or after chemotherapy. A VCD may not be recommended, however, if a man is taking medications to thin his blood or if some of his blood counts are abnormal. VCDs often work best for men who still achieve some swelling of the penis (i.e., a partial erection) with sexual excitement. Men who have very severe erection problems may not be able to get a completely firm or lasting erection with the device.

As you can see Figure 11.1, a VCD is a pump that a man places over his penis when he wants to have an erection. A number of companies manufacture VCDs. Some versions are pumped by hand, while others have a battery-powered pump. You pump the air out of the cylinder, creating a vacuum that draws blood into the shaft of the penis. The penis swells and becomes erect. If you take the pump off at that point, your erection will

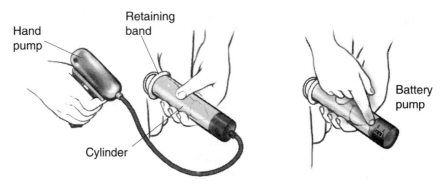

Figure 11.1 Vacuum constriction devices

soften. You load a *retaining band*—a rubber or plastic ring designed to be comfortable and easy to take off your penis—onto the pump before use. Once the pump has produced a firm erection, you slip the band down onto your penis. After you remove the pump, you will have an erection with a band around its base. You can leave the band on safely for up to half an hour to allow for successful intercourse. Some men say their VCD works best after they achieve a partial erection through foreplay. Other men, however, prefer to use the VCD before starting foreplay.

Using a VCD does not affect your ability to reach orgasm. If you were able to have an orgasm from sexual stimulation without the VCD, you should continue to reach one with VCD use. For about half of men, the retaining band is tight enough that it traps semen in the urethra during ejaculation. You would feel the pleasure of your orgasm, and you would not have any pain, but little or no semen would spurt out. The semen would drip out of your penis after you took the retaining band off.

The erection a VCD produces is often a bit thicker than a natural erection but is similar in length. The firmness is usually good, but it can vary. The penis may swivel more easily than normal where it joins the body. The erection also usually looks slightly blue or dusky in color and may feel cool to the touch. Some men keep a firm erection after orgasm, but, for many, the erection decreases at that point.

VCDs vary in cost from $300 to $500, depending on the brand and type. The battery-powered versions are generally more expensive, but they also may work a little more quickly. They are especially helpful for men who do not have good hand strength or coordination. Most insurance policies cover at least part of the costs of a VCD, especially if a medical cause for the erection problem has been documented.

About 50 percent to 80 percent of men are satisfied with a VCD, but others stop using it after a brief trial. In my experience, men who are in their midsixties or older and are in committed relationships are the ones most satisfied with a VCD. They typically feel glad to have an erection that works for intercourse and are not very concerned about having to wear the retaining band. (See Table 11.1 for advantages and disadvantages of the VCD.)

Douglas, a 76-year-old retired production supervisor, was undergoing chemotherapy for chronic leukemia. He had been widowed in his late fifties but had remarried Mamie, a woman he had known many years at work. Douglas and Mamie had a very happy life. After the shock of his diagnosis wore off, Douglas's biggest disappointment was that his erections deteriorated to the point that he and Mamie were unable to have intercourse. Douglas's first wife had died after years of battling colon cancer, so that their sex life had gone through a long, dormant period. Mamie's first husband was alcoholic and never very interested in sex. Douglas and Mamie valued the pleasure their sexual relationship had given to both of them.

When Douglas mentioned his sexual problem to his oncologist, he was referred to an impotence clinic at the same hospital where he was getting his cancer treatment. Of the options described, Douglas chose to try the vacuum pump. The first time he tried the pump, he and Mamie were both disappointed with the erection. It was not quite firm, and Douglas's penis kept slipping out during intercourse. He called up the information number of the company that made the device and was advised to practice getting an erection with it once a day outside of the sexual situation. After some practice, Douglas discovered the typical number of pumps it took to give him the best quality of erection. He also found out that he needed to wear a tighter retaining band to maintain the erection well. Mamie was very supportive of his efforts, and soon the couple was back to having regular lovemaking whenever Douglas felt well enough.

Penile Injections

Several medications can stimulate erections if you inject them with a needle directly into the side of your penis. Despite the mental image this evokes, most men say injecting is not particularly painful. A man can learn how to inject medication into the shaft of his own penis. Some men have their partners learn to do the injection. Most men use prostaglandin E1 (PGE1, or its trade name, Caverject) or a combination of papaverine and phentolamine (Regitine). Some men use a combination of all three drugs.

These drugs relax the smooth muscles within the penis, promoting blood flow. A combination of a low dose of medication plus the excitement and

Table 11.1
Advantages and Disadvantages of a Vacuum Constriction Device

Area of Concern	Advantages	Disadvantages
Risk of side effects	If used correctly, physical damage rarely occurs.	Should not keep band on for more than 30 minutes or fall asleep with the band on.
Number of office visits	One session to learn to use the device; some programs prescribe them with a teaching video only.	May need to return for more advice if VCD not working well; some manufacturers offer free advice by phone; a follow-up visit is a good idea.
Sexual pleasure	Better erection allows intercourse to take place and allows more relaxed foreplay.	May cause mild numbness or a cool sensation on the penis; the band can trap semen, producing a dry climax; erection may swivel at the base, limiting the positions for intercourse.
Problems with pain	Involves no surgery or needles.	Some men have mild discomfort during pumping or small black-and-blue marks on their skin after use; constriction bands can cause discomfort for some men.
Hassle quotient	None	Interrupts foreplay for several minutes.
Effect on fertility	May help penetration during intercourse.	Restriction of semen outflow makes this a poor choice for a man trying to father a child.
Effect on sexually transmitted diseases	Produces a firmer erection that aids condom use.	None
Impact on partner	Prolonging foreplay without worrying about losing an erection helps partner's satisfaction; erection may be slightly thicker with a VCD.	Some partners feel a VCD reduces the spontaneity of sex; may be embarrassing with a new partner.
Insurance coverage	A VCD is often affordable without insurance coverage; coverage is usually good.	No Medicaid coverage, at least in some states; most other insurers do cover.

physical stimulation of foreplay often produces a firm erection. The erection may last for a while even after ejaculation, becoming completely soft only when the medicine wears off.

In rare cases, the erection may stay firm for more than three hours. Then you must go to the emergency room so that a physician can inject special medication into your penis to reverse the erection. Otherwise, severe scarring in the penis can occur. If your physician prescribes a low dose of medication and you follow instructions carefully, the risk of prolonged erection is quite small. Your erections should last thirty to forty-five minutes at most. If they routinely last for an hour or two, the dose may be too high.

PGE1 injections often cause an aching or burning sensation in the penis for a few minutes. Some men have no pain at all, and others experience only mild discomfort. If pain is severe, it certainly can make injection therapy a less attractive option. Sometimes a small amount of local anesthetic is added to the prostaglandin medication to prevent pain. Other men switch to alternate medications or to a combination of drugs that includes only a low dose of PGE1.

Injections also may cause scar tissue to form in the penis. Most scarring does not affect a man's erections but feels like a small lump when a physician carefully examines the penis. In a minority of men, however, the scarring causes erections to become curved, making penetration for intercourse uncomfortable or even impossible. Once a curvature forms, it rarely goes away by itself. The only effective treatment is reconstructive surgery, often involving a penile prosthesis (see page 95 and pages 97–101). Some men have a tendency to form scar tissue in the penis even without using injections. This condition is called Peyronie's disease, and its symptoms are pain with erection and development of a penile curvature. It may be that injection therapy speeds up the scarring process in men at risk for Peyronie's disease. Unfortunately, there is no procedure for early identification of these men.

Some men with an anxiety-based erection problem use injections to gain self-confidence. Strong anxiety can override the effect of the injection, however, so that a man does not get a satisfactory erection. These men are often disappointed with injection therapy and just stop using it. Injection therapy is more successful in men who have poor circulation in the penis or who have erection problems due to nerve damage, for example, after radical pelvic cancer surgeries such as radical prostatectomy, cystectomy, or abdominoperineal resection.

Urology researchers at Boston University School of Medicine recently suggested that using PGE1 penile injections in the months after nerve-sparing pelvic surgery may increase a man's chance of recovering firm erections. Getting regular erections from injection therapy may prevent a natural substance called collagen from forming after surgery in the spongy tissue of the penis. Collagen deposits, which also form with aging, make the tissue of the penis less elastic. The chambers of the penis cannot relax and allow a firm erection to occur.

An Italian group recently compared men assigned to use penile injections of PGE1 three times a week starting a month after radical prostate surgery to men not given the medication. The injection group was more likely to recover useful erections by six months after surgery. Unfortunately, there is a catch: Researchers at the Cleveland Clinic found that a third of men have severe pain with prostaglandin injections in the first year after their pelvic cancer surgery, the period in which injection therapy is touted as a preventive measure. Pain problems do lessen with time, however.

If using injection therapy soon after surgery enhances recovery of erections, perhaps similar results could be achieved with less pain and risk by using a vacuum device regularly to increase blood flow to the penis. Is it the blood flow of erection or is it the PGE1 that prevents collagen deposits? The answer is not yet known.

A few men never achieve good erections with injection therapy, but most are successful after some adjustment of dose or type of medication. In general, perhaps a quarter to a half of men stop injection treatment for various reasons in the first year of using it.

The cost of injection therapy varies, depending on the type of medication used; but, in general, with medication and supplies (syringes, sterile wipes, etc.), the cost is somewhere around $50 to $100 per month. Injection medications usually are prescribed in a liquid form. Because the medications weaken after a few weeks or months, their containers are labeled with an expiration date, after which the medications may no longer be effective and should not be used. Caverject comes in powdered form, which extends its potency until it is mixed up for use. It also is more expensive, however. Insurance companies vary in their coverage for these prescriptions. (See Table 11.2 for advantages and disadvantages of injection therapy.)

Roger was only 47 when he had a radical prostatectomy. He had recently divorced and was dating a woman ten years younger. Of course sexual function was a strong concern for him. However, his surgeon was able to spare the nerves on only one side of the prostate gland because of the size of Roger's tumor. In the weeks after his operation, Roger noticed that he woke on some days with a partial erection that was not really firm. As soon as he felt well enough, he tried masturbation. He could reach orgasm, but his erection never got hard enough to allow for intercourse.

Roger's urologist instructed him in using Caverject. Roger was originally planning to inject himself in the bathroom before sex so that he would not have to tell his girlfriend about the problem. She was so supportive during his recovery from surgery, however, that he decided to trust her and be open about using injections. With the medication, he was able to get firm and lasting erections. He was a little frustrated that he was told not to use the medication more than twice a week because he and his partner had been having sex almost daily before his cancer was diagnosed. They compensated, though, by having lovemaking without penetration several nights a week.

Using Prostaglandin in the Urethra

Because many men hate the idea of injections, researchers have tried to find another way to get PGE1 into the cavernous bodies. The Muse system uses a suppository that you slip into your urethra using a special applicator. You or your partner rub your penis to help the medication spread through the mucous membrane of the urinary tube into the spongy tissue of the penis. An erection may begin after five to ten minutes. Some men still have burning pain after using the Muse system; and the other side effects of injection, such as prolonged erections and penile curvature, have also been seen with this treatment. It provides a good option for some men, but its effectiveness compared to injection is not yet clear.

Penile Prostheses

Penile prostheses are often called penile implants—not to be confused with a penile *transplant*. Even with modern medical technology, a man is stuck with the organ he received at birth! Early penile implants were rods made of silicone that were surgically placed in a man's penis to make it permanently erect. Today's penile prostheses can produce an erection that looks and feels much more natural. Some men still receive rod-type penile prostheses, but the rods are *malleable*: They have a bendable metal core so that a man can curve his penis and tuck it out of the way during normal activities and straighten it to the erect position for sex.

Most men now get inflatable penile prostheses (IPPs), which give a

Table 11.2
Advantages and Disadvantages of Injection Therapy

Area of Concern	Advantages	Disadvantages
Risk of side effects	No surgery needed.	About 10% to 15% of men develop scar tissue in penis after a year of use; scarring can cause erections to be permanently curved; there is a small risk of prolonged erections and emergency room visits.
Number of office visits	Several sessions are needed to learn injection technique and adjust the dose of medication.	Need to return to check every few months for scarring.
Sexual pleasure	Better erection allows intercourse to take place and allows more relaxed foreplay; no change in skin sensation.	None
Problems with pain	No surgery	A few men find the injection painful; about half have an ache in the penis after using PGE1, but the ache may fade in a few minutes and is tolerable to most.
Hassle quotient	Injection can be done before starting sex.	Need to be prepared to have sex by having equipment with you.
Effect on fertility	May improve penetration during intercourse.	None known
Effect on sexually transmitted diseases	Produces a firmer erection that aids condom use.	Bleeding at the injection site (which is rare) could theoretically add to the risk of transmitting or receiving sexually transmitted viruses; there is no current scientific evidence for such transmission.
Impact on partner	Being able to take time in foreplay without worrying about losing an erection helps partner's satisfaction.	Some partners feel injections reduce the spontaneity of sex; may be embarrassing with a new partner.
Insurance coverage	None	Insurance coverage varies; cost is ongoing rather than a one-time fee.

man the option of having an erect penis for sexual activity and a soft penis the rest of the time. Two companies, American Medical Systems and Mentor, manufacture these implants, and they come in self-contained, two-piece, or three-piece versions. Figure 11.2 shows the three types. The more complex the implant, the firmer and larger the erection it produces, and the more natural the soft state of the penis. On the other hand, the more parts in the implant, the more possibility of a mechanical breakdown over the years.

All IPPs share some features. They include two cylinders and a pump system surgically placed in the penis and surrounding pelvic area. To get an erection, a man must press on a small pump that transfers fluid into the cylinders in the penis. The penis does not deflate after orgasm until the man himself activates a release valve that is part of the device. Other people would probably not be able to tell that a man had an IPP, unless they spotted his small surgical scar, usually located where the bottom of the penis meets the scrotal sac. Men would not be embarrassed in a locker room or public rest room, for example.

An IPP does not change sensation on the skin of the penis or a man's ability to reach orgasm, nor does it affect ejaculation and urination. However, once a penile prosthesis is implanted, it destroys the natural erection reflex—if the implant is removed, the man will never again have natural erections. Therefore, a penile prosthesis is used only when there is a clear medical cause for the erection problem and when erections are unlikely to improve naturally. Surgery is not commonly used to treat stress-related erection problems that may get better with counseling or time. After can-

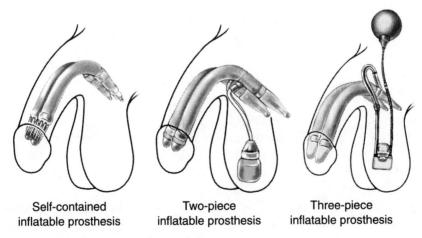

| Self-contained inflatable prosthesis | Two-piece inflatable prosthesis | Three-piece inflatable prosthesis |

Figure 11.2   Types of penile prosthesis

cer treatment, an IPP may be an excellent way of restoring erections. Men who have had radical pelvic surgery, however, such as radical prostatectomy or abdominoperineal resection, should wait for a long enough period (at least a year, and perhaps up to two years) to make sure their own erections will not recover before scheduling surgery to have an IPP. In the meanwhile, they can use a vacuum pump or penile injections.

The ideal penile prosthesis would produce a penis that looked and felt totally normal in the flaccid (soft) state and in the erect state. No prosthesis has yet reached this standard.

Self-Contained IPPs

The simplest IPPs are the self-contained models, consisting of two silicone cylinders that are implanted in the penis. Each cylinder contains its own pump system that uses air pressure to transfer fluid from a rear chamber to a front chamber. When the front chamber is empty, the penis is limp, though it may look larger than usual and feel less soft. To produce an erection, a man must squeeze pumps on the left and right sides located just behind the head of the penis. Fluid gets transferred to the front chamber of each cylinder, making the penis rigid. To deflate the IPP, a man bends his erection downward.

The erection is typically thinner and shorter than a full, natural erection, and a partner may be able to feel the cylinders in the shaft of the penis. Although the cylinders are made in several sizes, this type of IPP may not work well for a man whose penis is larger than most. The advantage is that the surgery is very brief and simple, and the surgeon does not have to enter the pelvic area where previous cancer surgery or radiation therapy may have caused scar tissue.

Two-Piece IPPs

Two-piece IPPs also have two cylinders that fit in the penis, but they are connected to a combination pump and reservoir that is placed in the loose skin of a man's scrotum, between his testicles. The separate reservoir can hold more fluid, creating a firmer and slightly larger erection when the implant is inflated. A man inflates his IPP by squeezing on the pump a few times through his skin. The pump is placed so that squeezing does not put uncomfortable pressure on the testicles. Pumping transfers fluid from the reservoir to the cylinders in the penis, inflating them. Pressing on a deflation valve at the base of the pump returns the fluid to the reservoir, deflating the penis. The erection from a two-piece IPP usually has good rigidity and thickness but will be shorter than a natural erection. Although the surgery is a little more complex than that to put in a self-contained IPP, it still avoids disturbing the pelvic area.

Three-Piece IPPs

The fanciest IPPs are the three-piece types. Two cylinders in the penis are connected by tubing to a separate reservoir that holds fluid and is tucked under the groin muscles. This type of reservoir can hold a greater amount of fluid to produce the fullest erection. A pump is also connected to the system, sitting in the scrotal sac between the testicles. When the penis is inflated, the three-piece IPP gives the penis stiffness and thickness that are very similar to a natural erection.

Some three-piece IPPs use cylinders that can also increase in length with inflation (the Ultrex IPP made by American Medical Systems), producing a longer erection. Even with these models, most men rate the erection as shorter than their previous normal penile length. Despite men's concern about penis length, most women are not upset if an erection becomes somewhat shorter. The sensitive part of a woman's vagina is its outer third, closest to the entrance. Even for women who regularly reach orgasm during intercourse, stimulation deep inside the vagina is less crucial than spending enough time on foreplay and thrusting. Many women reach orgasm most easily when they are on top during intercourse, a position that does not provide deep penetration but does give a woman the chance to maximize friction against the clitoris during intercourse.

If a man has had cancer surgery in the pelvis or radiation therapy to that area, putting in a three-piece IPP can be more risky. Routinely, the surgeon makes just one small incision and can place all the equipment inside the body from that opening. The reservoir, however, goes into the pelvis. If the surgeon tries to place the reservoir in the usual way—by blindly making a pocket for it from below—he may poke a hole through a piece of bowel that has gotten stuck in an unusual place because of previous cancer treatment. Then a temporary colostomy is necessary to prevent infection while the injury heals. An alternative procedure is to make a separate small incision for the reservoir so that the surgeon can see what he or she is doing during that part of the operation.

Another potential risk is putting the reservoir in an area of weakened tissue so that it would eventually rub through and get displaced. A man who has had previous pelvic cancer treatment may be safer choosing a simpler type of IPP.

Complications

One potential complication of having an IPP is mechanical failure. If part of the device springs a tiny leak, some of the internal fluid will be lost. Device failures rarely cause pain or damage a man's health. The only way to repair them, however, is to have another small surgery to replace the broken part.

A more serious problem occurs if an infection develops during the first few days after the implant surgery. The IPP is a foreign body and can act as a hiding place for bacteria. The only way to cure the infection is to remove the IPP, treat the infection with powerful antibiotics, and then wait several months before trying to put in a new IPP. Because infection typically causes scar tissue, the ultimate surgical result may not be as good as the original. Special precautions are taken to avoid infection when surgery for an IPP is planned, so only about 2 percent of men have surgical infections.

Once the area is healed after a successful transplant, a man should routinely have preventive antibiotics before certain medical procedures, such as having his teeth cleaned. This is to make sure that any bacteria that enter the bloodstream will never contaminate the IPP.

About 90 percent to 95 percent of IPP surgeries are successful; that is, the implants function well and produce usable erections. However, it is not known how many men have surgery and then are rarely sexually active. Typically 80 percent to 90 percent of men express satisfaction and say that they would choose surgery again. More detailed questions, however, suggest that some men who feel overall that they made the right choice still are dissatisfied with the appearance and size of the penis or their pleasure during sex. (See Table 11.3 for pros and cons of prostheses.)

The total professional and hospital fees for implanting an IPP vary, but they are usually between $15,000 and $20,000. Insurance coverage for these operations is usually good, as long as a medical cause of the erection problem has been documented, for example, by a urologist's examination and monitoring of sleep erections.

Table 11.3
Advantages and Disadvantages of an Inflatable Penile Prosthesis

Area of Concern	Advantages	Disadvantages
Risk of side effects	One-time surgery avoids risk of curvature of the penis or emergency room visits.	Infection during healing may require removal of implant in about 2% of cases; implants fail and another surgery is needed to replace a broken part in about 5% of cases in the first 5 years.
Number of office visits	Usually just one or two follow-up visits after surgery.	Surgery usually involves 2 or 3 days in hospital and time off from work.
Sexual pleasure	Better erection allows intercourse to take place and allows more relaxed foreplay; no change in skin sensation.	Some men feel that a shorter penis limits intercourse positions.
Problems with pain	Most men have no pain after about 6 weeks.	A few men have prolonged tenderness in the penis after surgery.
Hassle quotient	Takes less time to inflate implant than to use a VCD or an injection; can inflate before beginning sex; no external equipment needed.	If device ever fails, another surgery is needed to repair it.
Effect on fertility	May help improve penetration during intercourse.	None known
Effect on sexually transmitted diseases	Produces a firmer erection that aids condom use.	None, once healing is complete.
Impact on partner	Being able to prolong foreplay without worrying about losing an erection helps partner's satisfaction.	Some partners feel the device reduces the spontaneity of sex or is artificial; may be embarrassing with a new partner.
Insurance coverage	Usually good if a medical cause is documented.	Usually not covered if erection problem has no medical cause.

Sex Therapy for Erection Problems

If you have an anxiety-based erection problem, sex therapy may be helpful. When men have stress-related erection problems, sex therapy including their partner resolves the problem about 50 percent to 70 percent of the time. Success rates with the man alone in counseling are somewhat lower. If a man does not have a committed partner, sessions may focus on how to communicate about the sexual problem with someone new and begin a sexual relationship within a framework that minimizes anxiety. Sex therapy is most likely to fail when a man drops out of treatment after only one or two sessions. Dropping out of treatment is a common problem that may happen when a couple has poor communication or when coming for sessions is inconvenient as a result of time or money pressures.

Sexual counseling can be helpful in conjunction with medical or surgical treatment for an erection problem, to guide a couple in agreeing on a treatment, and to help them improve their sexual communication and lovemaking skills so that they can make better use of the man's improved erections.

In most cities, the cost of a session of sex therapy varies between $80 and $150, depending on the training of the therapist and the local cost of living. Obviously, the total expense will vary depending on the number of sessions needed.

If you are trying to figure out whether sex therapy could help, you can read about sex therapy exercises to overcome an anxiety-based erection problem in the book *The New Male Sexuality* (see Resources under Books). And see Table 11.4, which lays out the advantages and disadvantages of sex therapy.

Howard decided to have an inflatable penile prosthesis put in as soon as he knew he was going to have his bladder removed. A semiretired computer consultant, he believed you could rebuild a system and make it function almost like new. He was having his surgeon create a new bladder so that he would continue to urinate through his penis, and he had originally hoped the penile implant could be put in at the same time. However, his surgeon said that the operation would be complex and lengthy enough without adding that extra factor.

As the surgeon had predicted, Howard's erections did not recover after his radical cystectomy. Howard waited six months and asked the surgeon to schedule an operation to install a penile prosthesis. He was not interested in any other treatment because he wanted to feel that erections were generated internally. Although the surgery took place without a hitch, Howard and his

Table 11.4
Advantages and Disadvantages of Sex Therapy

Area of Concern	Advantages	Disadvantages
Risk of side effects	May improve the couple's general communication.	May highlight conflict in a relationship.
Number of office visits	Will be fewer if the couple does their homework.	Must return for a number of visits.
Sexual pleasure	Potential to have better sexual communication and skills than before therapy began.	None
Problems with pain	No physical pain	May bring up emotionally painful topics.
Hassle quotient	No artificial devices	Touching exercises involve teamwork and having sex in a new format.
Effect on fertility	May help men relax when asked to perform for infertility treatment.	Some phases of treatment involve postponing intercourse for several weeks.
Effect on sexually transmitted diseases	May help men feel more comfortable using condoms.	None
Impact on partner	When the partner is included, satisfaction with treatment is often increased.	Some partners are not willing to participate in sex therapy.
Insurance coverage	Short-term sex therapy may be affordable without insurance coverage.	Insurance coverage is often poor for counseling services; some policies exclude treatment for sexual dysfunction.

wife never resumed their sex life. Instead, Howard avoided coming to bed until his wife fell asleep. He had never been a man to give many hugs or compliments, but he became even more withdrawn.

When Howard returned for his yearly cancer follow-up, his wife asked to be present. Howard was a little miffed but was much more surprised and upset when his wife asked the surgeon point blank whether Howard was capable of having sex. The surgeon asked if there was a problem with the prosthesis. Howard's wife said she had never even seen her husband undressed since his surgery.

Howard sat red-faced and silent. He finally explained that he did not think it was worth trying sex with the erection he could get—it had decreased from being six and seven-eighths inches to only five. He did not believe he could satisfy his wife now. Howard's wife responded angrily that she had never measured her husband's penis with a ruler to see if it were long enough. If he was not interested in sex, however, she at least would appreciate a back rub or a hug.

Howard hung his head. He had always had an easier time with programming than with conversation. The surgeon knew he was out of his depth, but he did get Howard and his wife to agree to see a sex therapist. Howard was quite uncomfortable with the idea of counseling, but he was able to see the value of structured exercises to do at home. Howard's wife had long ago stopped expecting romance from her husband, but she was gratified to have some physical contact with him again. And Howard discovered that sexual communication was a kind of "software" to make his new "hardware" more user-friendly.

Finding the Treatment That Works for You

Sometimes your doctor will steer you to a particular treatment for an erection problem. A man in very poor health, for example, may want something simple and safe, like a VCD. A man whose problem is clearly stress-related should explore sex therapy as an option because a successful treatment will give him skills he can use for the rest of his life and does not risk damaging his healthy penis. For many men, particularly those with a medical cause for their erection problem, the choice of treatment depends on individual preferences. If you are married or in a committed relationship, sharing this chapter with your partner and discussing the choices can be helpful.

As you may notice from the success rates quoted, none of the treatments works for everyone. If you try a treatment and are dissatisfied, let your doctor know. Perhaps a different treatment would be more acceptable than you thought at first. Unfortunately, many men give up after trying one treatment and never come back to explain what went wrong. Try making a list of your concerns and what it would take to make you happy with another treatment. Be sure to discuss your dissatisfaction with your partner, too. You may think she is upset about a change in your erection and find that it really is not an issue for her.

Now we will turn our attention from the arousal phase of sex to its climax. The next chapter reviews how cancer can interfere with both men's and women's ability to reach orgasm.

12

The Bells Aren't Ringing: No Orgasms, Slow Orgasms, and Dry Orgasms

Cancer treatment can change your capacity to reach orgasm in several ways. You may take a long time to reach orgasm, need stronger stimulation, or be unable to have an orgasm at all. If you are a man, you may have a dry orgasm, without ejaculating any semen.

No Orgasms or Slow Orgasms

It is actually fairly unusual to develop a new problem with reaching orgasm as a result of cancer treatment. At the sexual rehabilitation clinic at the University of Texas M. D. Anderson Cancer Center in Houston, problems with orgasm were the least common reason that men or women asked for help.

Your ability to reach orgasm depends on having normal skin sensation in the erotic zones of your body. The nerves that help you feel pleasure when your genital skin is caressed are rarely damaged by cancer treatment because they hug the side walls of the pelvis and are protected by a tough layer of tissue. Treatment for tumors of the brain or spinal cord can sometimes lead to paralysis and numbness, similar to the impact of a stroke or a spinal cord injury. In that case, pleasure from genital touch may be lost, though you can still enjoy sexual fantasies and learn to focus on erotic pleasure when areas with normal sensation are touched.

Other people have surgery to remove an important genital area, such as the penis or vulva. Amazingly, many still feel pleasure on the skin that is left and learn how to reach orgasm again from sexual fantasies or caressing (see Chapter 25). In a similar way, after mastectomy, women usually can compensate for the loss of pleasurable breast caressing.

A mild loss of genital sensation is more common after cancer treatment and can increase the time or effort it takes to reach orgasm. We know that men experience some loss of skin sensitivity on the penis just with normal aging, and similar changes may occur for women after menopause. When cancer treatment leaves a man or woman with low androgen levels, pleasure with sexual touch often decreases. High doses of some types of chemotherapy, especially those containing platinum, cause damage to nerves. The usual result is numbness or tingling in hands and feet, but occasionally someone has mentioned to me noticing some lost sensitivity on the genital area as well.

Medications That Interfere with Orgasm

If reaching orgasm is your main sexual problem, a medication could be the culprit, particularly if you are taking one of the newer antidepressant drugs. The serotonin reuptake inhibitors, including the drugs Prozac, Paxil, and Zoloft, delay orgasm so often that they are currently being used to treat men who complain of premature ejaculation. Unfortunately, most women do not want to take a longer time to reach orgasm, and antidepressants can also prevent orgasm completely for women or men who need higher doses. Tranquilizers also can interfere with reaching orgasm, as can high doses of narcotic pain medication.

Strategies for Reaching Orgasm More Easily

If you are finding it a chore to reach orgasm or if you are unable to have one since your cancer treatment, here are some strategies to try:

- Focus on increasing your desire and arousal instead of straining to reach orgasm. If sex feels intensely pleasurable, you will eventually climax. (See Chapter 9 for suggestions.)

- If you are taking so long to reach orgasm that sex is becoming a chore for you or your partner, change your goals. Try making sex as much fun as possible, without worrying about orgasms. If you do not have one in a reasonable period of time, quit for that day. Having sex without an orgasm will not harm your health.

• It may be easier to learn to reach orgasm again by using your own self-stimulation. When you are alone, you do not have to worry about your partner's getting tired, and you receive immediate feedback when you try different types of touching. Once you can reach orgasm in masturbation, you can teach your partner what works.

• A vibrator can help because it provides a strong and steady kind of stimulation. You do not have to worry that your vibrator is getting tired or bored (although it can be a letdown when the batteries go dead—keep some spares handy)! Unique nerves in the skin that sense vibration sometimes remain intact when an illness has damaged the nerves sensing light touch.

If the idea of a vibrator sounds impersonal and mechanical, imagine using it as part of playful lovemaking with your partner. For women, vibrators usually work best when moved lightly around the area of the clitoris, varying the pressure and the location from moment to moment. Fewer women find vibrators pleasurable when used inside the vagina. For a man, a vibrator often gives pleasure when it is moved around on the sensitive head of the penis. Some vibrators have cup-shaped attachments for men that transmit vibration to the entire head of the penis. You can hold a small vibrator against the base of the penis to provide extra sensation during intercourse.

Look for a vibrator that is quiet and has more than one speed, so that you can try it on low or high. The best vibrators are usually not the penis-shaped ones advertised in adult bookstores. Rather they are sturdier models meant to be used for nonsexual massaging as well as sexual stimulation. Some are shaped like a wand and have a soft, cylindrical vibrating head at the top. Others have a handle with several attachments that snap onto a vibrating shaft (see the Resources under Products to Enhance Sex).

When James had an abdominoperineal resection for colon cancer, he and his wife had been married for 42 years. After surgery, James was extremely frustrated to find that he could not get a firm erection during foreplay. After a few minutes of caressing from his wife, he would take her hand off of his penis and say, "It's no use." Every couple of months, she would snuggle up to James and try to get him interested in lovemaking, but always with the same result.

When James and his wife came to see me, I asked about their foreplay before cancer surgery. Had they spent much time on kissing and touching then? James's wife said that they had, but usually foreplay meant James caressing her. He was uncomfortable when she tried to caress his penis because he feared it would make him climax too quickly. James's wife was open to trying more caressing, however, and even offered to experiment with some oral sex or a vibrator.

I asked the couple to experiment with touch, but without any expectation that it would result in an erection, intercourse, or orgasms. After several tries, James reported that he could reach an orgasm. He still ejaculated semen and felt the intensity was satisfying. Eventually, his erections improved and the couple was able to return to having intercourse.

Premature Ejaculation after Cancer

One piece of good news is that cancer and its treatments do not cause premature ejaculation, a problem in which men reach climax very rapidly, either before they can penetrate for intercourse or within a minute or two afterward. Premature ejaculation is the most common sexual problem among young men, one that often lessens with age and sexual experience. It is not a medical problem, however, and can be better described as a bad habit or a failure to learn how to last longer. The book *The New Male Sexuality* contains a self-help guide to overcoming premature ejaculation (see Resources under Books).

Dry Orgasms: Where Is the Semen?

A variety of cancer therapies leave a man with dry orgasms. He experiences the pleasure of orgasm and the muscles at the base of the penis pump rhythmically, but no semen comes out of his penis. See Table 12.1 for the types of treatments that can cause this.

Damage to the Semen Factory

The prostate and seminal vesicles manufacture seminal fluid. They are removed as part of several radical pelvic surgeries, including radical prostatectomy, radical cystectomy, and total pelvic exenteration. Men who have these operations typically have erection problems but can reach orgasm with hand caressing or oral sex. What do these orgasms feel like? Interviews with men who had surgery for bladder cancer revealed that about half said their climax felt pleasurable, but weaker than normal.

Table 12.1
Cancer Treatments That Cause Dry Orgasm

Type of Treatment	Reason for Dry Orgasm
Radical prostatectomy	Prostate and seminal vesicles are removed.
Radical cystectomy	Prostate and seminal vesicles are removed.
Pelvic radiation therapy	Prostate and seminal vesicles are damaged.
Retroperitoneal lymphadenectomy	Nerves that control emission are damaged.
Abdominoperineal resection or sigmoidectomy	Nerves that control emission are damaged.
Some chemotherapy drugs	Nerves that control emission are damaged.

Another large group of men said their climax felt about the same as before surgery. About 10 percent of the men reported that their orgasms were better than in the past—more pleasurable and longer lasting.

Radiation therapy to the pelvis can damage the prostate and seminal vesicles so much that they produce little or no semen. After radiation therapy for prostate cancer, men often have dry orgasms. Men who have radiation therapy for seminoma also sometimes report ejaculating only a few drops of semen.

Damage to Emission Control

Remember from Chapter 2 that men's orgasms have two stages: In the first stage, emission, the prostate and seminal vesicles squeeze out the semen, and the valve to the bladder shuts tightly. If either of these processes does not take place, a man will have a dry orgasm once the second stage of orgasm, ejaculation, begins.

The nerve pathway that controls emission can be damaged during cancer surgery. Some colorectal cancer operations can damage sympathetic nerves that lie between the lower spinal cord and the colon. Another operation that often interrupts this pathway, but higher up in the body, is *retroperitoneal lymphadenectomy* (removal of lymph nodes to decide whether chemotherapy is needed for men who have testicular cancer). Some chemotherapy drugs themselves are occasionally reported to cause dry orgasm.

How does the nerve damage cause dry orgasm? If the damage is severe, the prostate and seminal vesicles are paralyzed and do not squeeze out their fluids. This is called *failure of emission*. Some men have dry orgasms but with a less severe change. The muscle tissue of the prostate and seminal vesicles is not paralyzed, but a valve (called the internal sphincter) between the bladder and prostate does not shut correctly during orgasm. As a result, semen spurts backward into the bladder, a problem called *retrograde ejaculation*.

Whether dry orgasm is caused by failure of emission or retrograde ejaculation, the results feel the same. Most men say their orgasm is just as pleasurable as always, but perhaps a quarter of men feel that some of the sensation is missing. Men sometimes worry that dry orgasm deprives a woman of pleasure, but most women do not feel semen spurting into the vagina during intercourse. In fact, many women say that dry orgasm is an improvement because they feel more comfortable giving a man oral sex and do not have semen dripping out of their vaginas after intercourse!

If a man would still like to father a child, dry orgasm becomes a big problem, however. The sperm cells have no way to get into the vagina. Several medical treatments are available and will be discussed in Chapter 18 when we focus on infertility after cancer.

13

Causes of Painful Sex

Pain during sex is one of the most common problems women experience after cancer treatment, although it is a less frequent issue for men.

Chronic Pain That Interferes with Sex

It is hard to get in the mood for sex if cancer treatment leaves you with chronic pain, even if the area that hurts is outside the pelvis. After cancer treatment, some men or women have pain where an arm or leg had to be amputated or in a place where cancer has spread to the bone. Chronic pain causes fatigue and irritability, and, as was mentioned in Chapter 8, pain medications also can decrease sexual desire. Pain that is centered on the genital area is even more problematic for sex.

Pain in the Genital Area for Women

Cancer treatments can lead to genital pain for women in several different ways.

Pain Related to Menopause

Whether cancer treatment brings on a premature and sudden menopause or if a woman was already menopausal but cannot risk using estrogen replacement after cancer (see Chapter 3), she may have trouble with vaginal dryness and tightness during penetration and intercourse and with burning or soreness after sex. Loss of stretch in the vaginal tissues can also make deep penetration uncomfortable. Urinary tract or yeast infections, more frequent after menopause, make intercourse painful.

Pain Related to Pelvic Radiation Therapy

Radiation therapy directed at the vagina, as in treatment for vaginal or cervical cancer, can lead to pain with sex. The lining of the vagina becomes very irritated toward the end of radiotherapy; and, without special preventive treatment, the vaginal walls can actually stick together, closing up the vagina as healing takes place. A few women develop vaginal ulcers, areas in which the radiation damages the vaginal lining so much that an open sore forms. Ulcers are painful and take weeks to heal.

In a gradual process that may continue over several years after treatment, the walls of the vagina develop tough scar tissue. The vagina may appear generally smaller, or sometimes tight rings of scar tissue form in one particular area of the vaginal canal.

Much radiation damage to the vagina can be prevented by making sure the vaginal canal is opened and the muscular walls of the vagina are stretched regularly during the healing process. This exercise to the vagina prevents tight scar tissue from forming but may be painful soon after treatment, when irritation is still strong. Penile-vaginal sexual intercourse is one natural way of preventing scarring. For women who are not having intercourse with a male partner, an alternative is to use vaginal dilators (see Chapter 14).

Pain after Bone Marrow Transplant

Scar tissue can also form in the vagina after bone marrow transplant, either if radiation to the whole body is used to kill a woman's bone marrow before the transplant or if the marrow comes from a donor and graft versus host disease develops.

Pain during Chemotherapy

Chemotherapy drugs that cause *mucositis* (a very painful irritation of the lining of the mouth) can also cause vaginal irritation. Oncologists often do not realize that these side effects occur, or else they fail to warn women about them. Vaginal irritation usually clears up after several days, but it will reoccur if the same irritating chemotherapy drug is given. Often, women who have been exposed to the virus that causes genital herpes have more frequent or severe outbreaks of painful genital blisters during chemotherapy because the immune system is temporarily depressed (see Chapter 6).

Pain Related to Surgical Scarring

Cancer surgery that removes part of the vulva or vagina can leave painful scar tissue or can reduce the size of the vagina (see Chapter 25). Operations that remove pelvic organs, such as the rectum or uterus, also can create *adhesions* (filmy scar tissue that sticks inner organs together). Sexual activity, particularly deep thrusting of the penis during intercourse, can pull on the adhesions and causes pain deep in the vagina. Occasionally, an ovary left in place after a hysterectomy gets stuck to the top of the vagina during healing. Because the ovary is quite sensitive, it hurts if thrusting hits against it. If the rectum is removed, women may find that some intercourse positions are painful because of the loss of cushioning in the area behind the rear vaginal wall.

Finding the Cause of the Pain

If the cause of a woman's genital pain is not obvious, a thorough pelvic examination by a concerned and expert gynecologist may help. An examination for pain should include very careful inspection of the vulva. Sometimes the gynecologist will touch a cotton swab to different areas to locate places that are especially tender. If a woman has burning pain or severe tenderness right around the vaginal entrance, a *colposcopy* (looking at the vulva through a special microscope) may help identify chronic inflammation, called *vulvar vestibulitis*, that is not obvious to the naked eye. A colposcopy can also help diagnose precancerous and malignant changes on the skin of the vulva, although these are usually not painful.

In women who have had pelvic surgery or radiotherapy, the gynecologist should evaluate whether the vaginal entrance has become tightened by scar tissue and whether vaginal depth and width and stretchiness of the vaginal tissues are normal. When women are in menopause, the exam can gauge whether a loss of estrogen has made the vaginal lining thin and fragile or has contributed to loss of vaginal size. A sample of cells from the vaginal lining can be analyzed to see if enough estrogen is present (maturation index).

For women who have pain deep in the pelvic area during the thrusting of intercourse, the gynecologist can try to reproduce the painful sensations during the examination by using a finger to press on the upper vagina or to move the cervix. An ultrasound machine can be used to obtain a picture of the internal pelvic organs. Occasionally, a *laparoscopy* (an operation through a small incision in the navel, allowing the surgeon to see the inside of the pelvis through a special, lighted telescope) may be useful. During laparoscopy, sources of pain such as deposits of *endometriosis* (abnormal tissue that has migrated out from the lining of the uterus) or adhesions can be removed using heat or laser treatments.

Genital Pain in Men

Having pain during sex is not a common problem among men, but it does occasionally happen as a result of cancer treatment. Most commonly, pain occurs at the moment of ejaculation and may be centered on the urethra, the tip of the penis, or the area behind the scrotum and in front of the anus. After pelvic cancer surgery, some men notice chronic achiness around the scrotum. Sometimes the cause of the pain is obvious, for example, irritation in the urethra after chemotherapy is instilled into the bladder to treat bladder cancer. Often, however, the pain is difficult to diagnose or treat. As in women, adhesions may form inside the pelvis after surgery or radiation therapy. During the muscle contractions of orgasm, these adhesions get pulled and cause pain.

Some men experience pain in the urethra or penis with erection. This occurs sometimes if scar tissue in the penis is forming, causing a man's erection to curve. This condition is called Peyronie's disease. It is not usually related to cancer treatment but may be more common if men have had repeated cystoscopies to examine the inside of their bladder or if they have had radiation therapy to the penis. The pain typically subsides after several months, but the curvature remains and can only be corrected with surgery.

14

Overcoming Pain during Sex

In this chapter I suggest ways to minimize interference from pain in your sex life.

Sex and Coping with Chronic Pain after Cancer

Chronic pain during or after cancer treatment can certainly interfere with your sex life. If you can manage to get in the mood for sex, however, making love may actually distract you from aches and pains. Research suggests that when women become sexually excited through vaginal stimulation, pain sensations elsewhere in the body are dulled. What are some strategies to get in the mood for sex despite chronic pain?

• You may get temporary pain relief if you prepare for sex by using a transcutaneous electrical stimulation (TENS) unit (a machine that uses electrical pulses to the skin around the painful area to decrease pain sensation); taking a warm bath or shower to ease stiffness; doing stretching or other physical therapy exercises; or using imagery, meditation, or deep muscle relaxation.

• Try lovemaking at times of day when you are rested and your pain level is lowest, even if these are not the traditional times to have sex.

• Time your pain medication to be in effect when you are going to try sexual activity.

• Use the techniques from Chapter 9 to enhance your desire for sex and give an extra edge to your mood. If pain distracts you during sex, try to mentally refocus your attention on pleasurable feelings in your body, or see if you can lose yourself in a sexual fantasy.

Sol's prostate cancer had gradually advanced into his bones. He was taking hormones, but he had many days when he was tired and achy. He still could get in the mood to enjoy sex on a good day, and his wife, Candace, did all she could to make conditions right. She would spend a long time caressing his penis or giving him oral stimulation and even suggested that they watch an erotic video together. Sol was able to use a vacuum device to get a good erection for intercourse. Because Sol had a number of sore spots, he no longer had intercourse in positions that required him to support his weight on his arms or knees. Instead, Candace sat on top of him, while he leaned back against a big pillow shaped like the top of an armchair. She did most of the thrusting during intercourse, but that had always been the type of position that made it easiest for her to reach orgasm. Sol and Candace found times early in the day to try sex because by evening, Sol was usually exhausted.

Coping with Genital Pain for Women

Women can try a variety of strategies to prevent or minimize genital pain during sex.

Medications for Genital Pain

Genital pain is difficult to treat with pain medication. It is impractical for most women to use narcotic pain relievers before sex. You may not always know when you will make love, and pain medication takes more than a few minutes to get its full effect. Narcotics also tend to decrease sexual desire. Nonnarcotic pain relievers rarely seem very effective in dulling genital pain during sex. Although antidepressants can interfere with sexual function, they have been useful to treat chronic pain in the pelvic area. They also can soothe some of the burning, tingling pain of *neuropathies* (a pain that results from messages misfiring in the nervous system). Women sometimes develop vulvar burning related to neuropathy after chemotherapy or genital surgery. If your doctor prescribes an antidepressant, remember that it can take a couple of weeks for the medication to reach its full effectiveness. You need to take the medication regularly, not just when you are in pain. Often, the dose or type of antidepressant needs adjusting before you get the best pain relief possible.

If the pain you have during sex is related to a tender area on your skin surface, you may want to ask your doctor to prescribe some Xylocaine gel, which contains a mild numbing agent. Women often say that the gel burns when they first apply it to the vulva or vaginal entrance. After several minutes, however, sensation is reduced. Xylocaine gel has limits to its effectiveness: The pain relief wears off fairly quickly, and this medication cannot combat pain that arises from deeper in the tissue. Men may find that the gel numbs the penis slightly during intercourse. If this is a problem, the man can use a condom to avoid contact with the gel.

Unless you have had breast cancer, remember that pain related to menopausal vaginal changes is quickly reversed by estrogen replacement, whether in a vaginal cream, a pill, or a patch. Women with cancer may occasionally be offered other hormonal vaginal creams containing corticosteroids (cortisone creams) or androgens (testosterone cream). These salves can sometimes soothe irritation on the delicate skin of the vulva and around the vaginal entrance. Sometimes the creams burn on application, but the hope is that over several weeks they will help heal and thicken the outer layer of skin.

Vaginal Lubricants: The Inside Scoop

For women with vaginal dryness or very sensitive vulvar skin, using an extra lubricant for sexual activity is often a key to reducing pain. The lubricant you choose should be water-based. It should not be a lubricant that contain oils or petroleum jelly (e.g., Vaseline). It should not be perfumed because scents are one of the most common irritants on the delicate, genital tissue.

Your partner can use a gel lubricant when he caresses your vulva or vagina with his fingers. Keep your lubricant next to you when you make love so that you do not have to stop to go and get it. Putting on a lubricant can become a routine part of your lovemaking. Ask your partner to spread it around your clitoris and vaginal entrance during foreplay. Spread some over the head of his penis when you are caressing him. Before penetration for intercourse, both the penis and the vaginal entrance should be lubricated to minimize friction and tightness.

Women are often reluctant to use an extra lubricant for sexual activity. Here are some common reasons women give and some counterarguments:

- "A lubricant is not natural." It is not natural to have a vagina that has lost its own ability to lubricate and expand because of menopause.

Using a lubricant restores the vagina to the state that nature intended for sexual activity.

- "Lubricants are unhealthful and will give me infections." Water-based lubricants that do not contain perfumes or other irritants are not unhealthful. In fact, products like Replens (see Resources under Products to Enhance Sex) that restore a good pH to the vagina help to prevent infection. Even using a gel lubricant can prevent the vaginal and urinary tract irritation after sex that promotes infections in women after menopause.

- "Stopping to use a lubricant ruins the spontaneity of sex." Replens is designed to be used three times weekly at bedtime, not during sex. And using a gel lubricant can become part of your lovemaking. You and your partner can keep the lubricant next to the bed and just spread gel with your fingers around the genital area during foreplay.

- "My partner says the lubricant makes me too wet." If you have become menopausal because of your cancer treatment, it is unlikely that lubricants will create too much moisture. Perhaps this was a problem in the past.

- "We enjoy oral sex and the lubricants taste bad." Many lubricants today are made to be tasteless, and some are even flavored.

Gel lubricants are commonly available in drugstores without a prescription. One of the most effective gel lubricants, Astroglide, is not carried widely in stores but can be mail-ordered from catalogs (see Resources under Products to Enhance Sex).

Some women need lubrication inside the vagina, especially if they are menopausal or have had vaginal radiotherapy or reconstruction. In my experience, the most effective product for internal lubrication is Replens (see Resources under Products to Enhance Sex). Marketed as a vaginal moisturizer, Replens is meant to be used three times a week before bedtime. A woman inserts the gel into her vagina using a tampon-shaped applicator. Replens helps the vaginal lining retain moisture. One study showed that after twelve weeks of regular Replens use, women who were in menopause had vaginal examinations similar to those of women taking estrogen. Replens improved the vagina's moisture, stretchiness, and acidity. Besides making intercourse more comfortable, these changes could potentially help to prevent monilial infections. Some women dislike Replens because it increases their vaginal discharge. The amount of discharge tends to decrease after the first two weeks of use, however, so it is important to give the product a chance. Replens is sold over the counter, without a prescription, but it is more expensive than other lubricants—costing somewhere around twenty dollars a month. Women who have severe vaginal dryness and discomfort may want to use Replens regularly and supplement with a gel lubricant at the time of lovemaking.

Avoiding Vaginal Infections

Vaginal infections with fungal organisms or bacteria are a common source of genital pain that can occur during or after cancer treatment. Yeast organisms (monilia) are often present in small numbers in the vagina. To prevent monilia from multiplying, keep the vaginal area dry: Wear cotton underwear. If you wear pantyhose, use brands that have a cotton crotch insert. Avoid tight jeans. If you wear exercise gear, get cotton tights and leotards rather than synthetic fabrics that do not breathe. Change clothes as soon as you are finished working out. Do not sit around in a wet swimsuit.

Some women are sensitive to colored dyes in underwear or toilet paper and should use only white products. Avoid any perfumed vaginal sprays, douches, or even bubble baths, and do not use deodorant tampons or menstrual pads.

If you have vaginal itching, burning, or discharge, have your doctor take a culture rather than using over-the-counter antiyeast medications. These vaginal creams and suppositories can be irritating themselves. They work on the most common type of vaginal infection—monilia—but not on other types. It is especially important during cancer treatment, when your immune system may be suppressed, to know what kind of fungus or bacteria is responsible for a vaginal infection.

Avoiding Urinary Tract Infections and Irritation

Urinary tract infections (UTIs) also make intercourse painful. UTIs occur more often in women than in men because women have a shorter urethra (the tube from the bladder to the outside). A UTI typically occurs when bacteria that normally live in the intestinal system travel up the urethra and start to grow in the warm, wet tropical atmosphere of the bladder. Having sexual intercourse, and possibly using a diaphragm for contraception, can increase the risk of a UTI. During thrusting, bacteria get a boost up into the urethra, and any irritation of the area from sexual activity, especially in a woman who is menopausal, makes infection more likely.

Symptoms of infection include sharp pain during urination, especially as the bladder is almost finished emptying, a feeling of needing to urinate very frequently or urgently, and blood in the urine. If infection is severe or involves the kidneys, you may also run a fever or have back or side pain. If you have any symptoms of a UTI, especially during cancer treatment, you should alert your doctor immediately. A urine culture can identify the bacterial infection and help determine which antibiotic to prescribe. Women who have one UTI after another can take a low dose of antibiotics on a preventive basis, either daily or after having intercourse.

Similar urinary symptoms can occur without an infection, as a result of irritation during chemotherapy or pelvic radiation therapy. These problems are not as easy to treat as an infection, and pain may take longer to resolve. Having sex less frequently, keeping movement gentle, using lots of lubrication, trying different intercourse positions, or avoiding vaginal penetration altogether may give you some relief.

Relaxing Your Pelvic Floor Muscles

Tension in the muscles that surround the vaginal entrance, a problem called *vaginismus*, is a common factor in pain during sexual activity. Vaginismus can become a conditioned reflex if a woman experiences pain on resuming sex after cancer. Her muscles tense automatically whenever anything is at her vaginal entrance because she fears that penetration will hurt. Even when the physical damage that caused the pain has healed, the muscle spasm remains, like a child flinching away from the unlit stove after being burned.

You can learn how to control these muscles, however. The pubococcygeal (PC) muscle surrounds the outer third of the vaginal canal, closest to the entrance. It is connected to a sheet of muscle that also includes the on/off valves for urination and bowel movements. Once you know how to tighten your PC muscle, you can recognize the contrasting sensation when it is relaxed. Then you can practice relaxing the muscle.

Next time that you urinate, notice the squeezing motion you use when you want to shut off the flow of urine. Try the squeeze when you are not urinating but just sitting or lying comfortably. Can you feel a tensing at the entrance of your vagina? Even after pelvic cancer surgery, most women have voluntary control over the PC muscle. If your cancer treatment damaged your spinal cord, however, you may not be able to squeeze the muscle at will.

To check that you are tensing the right muscle, put a water-based lubricant on the tip of your finger or on a tampon with a rounded plastic applicator. (Playtex tampons work well.) Lie back on your bed or sit against some pillows with your knees up and apart. Hold the lubricated finger or tampon at the entrance to your vagina. If you are unsure of the exact location of the vaginal entrance, look at yourself in a hand mirror, for example, a lighted makeup mirror. You can use the diagram of the vulva in Chapter 3 as a guide. It may be easier to see if you use your hands to gently spread the inner lips apart. Try to squeeze the PC muscle and then let it go loose. When you feel the muscle is relaxed, slip just the lubricated tip of the finger or tampon into your vagina. Hold it there and try squeezing the PC muscle again. You should be able to feel your vagina move a little, gently squeezing on the finger or tampon. The PC muscle only surrounds the outer inch or two of your vagina. The deeper part of the vagina cannot squeeze voluntarily.

Once you have found your PC muscle, practice squeezing and relaxing it daily. These exercises are called *Kegels*, after the gynecologist who invented them, Arnold Kegel. You can do Kegels almost anytime—in the shower, while watching TV, or during lunch. Try to make Kegels a part of your daily routine, twice a day. There are several ways to do Kegels, but this method is easy to remember: Squeeze the PC muscle while you count to three, and then let it relax as loosely as you can. Do ten Kegels in a row. It only takes a couple of minutes to do ten Kegels, but practicing can help you learn to feel the difference between tension and relaxation in your PC muscle.

Some sex therapists believe that Kegels strengthen the PC muscle and help women reach orgasm more easily. There is little scientific evidence for this view, but Kegels certainly will not hurt you! They may enhance your sexual pleasure by making you more aware of pleasant feelings in your vagina. Men and women sometimes enjoy the sensation of a woman squeezing her PC muscle during intercourse.

Vaginal Dilators: A Treatment for Several Seasons

If you have been having troublesome pain during intercourse, and lubricants and muscle relaxation have not helped, you may want to work with a set of vaginal dilators. *Before you try using a vaginal dilator, check with your gynecologist to make sure you do not have a medical problem that a dilator could aggravate, especially if you have had radiation therapy or surgery in your pelvic or genital area.* Vaginal dilators are latex or plastic cylinders made in a range of sizes. Sets of dilators are made by a company called Milex in Chicago, but they can only be obtained with a physician's prescription and are fairly expensive. They are made of a soft latex rubber material that can be cleaned easily and vary from about the size of a finger to the size of an erect penis.

Some gynecologists suggest substituting plastic test tubes or tops from syringes of different sizes. Some women also have used vibrators or penis-shaped sex toys from adult bookstores or mail-order catalogs because they are typically made in several sizes, including small ones (see Resources under Products to Enhance Sex). If you try any dilator other than one prescribed by a physician, make sure it is clean, has not been used by anyone else, is not made of a material that can break easily, has no sharp or pointed edges, and is not larger than an erect penis would be.

Using Dilators to Promote Vaginal Muscle Relaxation

If painful sex has resulted in chronic tension in the vaginal muscles, a woman can practice relaxing while slipping in a very small dilator. As she builds her muscle relaxation skills, she can graduate to a larger dilator. In most cases, the goal is not to physically enlarge the vagina with the dilator, but rather to learn better control over the vaginal muscles.

Using Dilators after Radiation Therapy to the Vagina

When the vagina receives a dose of radiation therapy, a woman should use a vaginal dilator or have intercourse during and after the course of treatment to help the vagina stay flexible and open. Many programs suggest either having sexual intercourse or using a dilator for a total of at least three times a week, not only during radiotherapy, but for several years afterward. In fact, it may be important for the rest of a woman's life to either stay sexually active or use a dilator regularly. The dilators usually handed out in radiation therapy clinics are hard plastic cylinders with a rounded tip. A small, medium, or large is chosen, depending on the size of the woman's vaginal canal.

Some women have no intention of resuming intercourse after cancer treatment, or they may enjoy a lovemaking routine that does not include penile penetration of the vagina. Even so, they should follow the program of vaginal dilation recommended by their radiotherapist. After treatment for cancer of the cervix or vagina, it is crucial to be able to examine the vagina and make sure no cancer has returned. If the vagina shrinks severely, a good examination may not be possible or may cause intense pain.

> Claudia had radiation therapy for cervical cancer. She had been brought up in a strict Catholic household. Once her mother had found Claudia, as a small child, with her hand in her pants. Claudia had been spanked with a belt and told never to touch her genitals. In the years since, she had obeyed this rule and never touched or looked at her vulva unless she had a medical problem. Claudia's husband was the only sexual partner she had ever had. His idea of lovemaking was rather limited, and Claudia was uncomfortable anyway with caressing on her genitals. He had divorced her and married another woman several years before her cancer was diagnosed. Once her husband was gone, Claudia did not miss sex at all.
>
> Claudia's cancer diagnosis and treatment were especially traumatic for her because she hated having pelvic examinations and medical procedures involving her vagina. Her worst day was when the nurse in radiotherapy gave her a vaginal dilator, saying simply, "Here is a dilator. Put this jelly on it and put it inside your vagina three times a week. Hold it in for at least fifteen minutes." Claudia just nodded her head. At home she took the dilator out of the box. It looked like a white, waxy candle without a wick. It reminded her of whispered stories she had heard as a teenager about nuns using candles to masturbate. She threw the dilator into the garbage. When the nurse asked her on follow-up visits if she was using the dilator, Claudia always said, "Oh certainly."
>
> Although Claudia's cancer did not return, her follow-up pelvic examinations became very painful and difficult. Her gynecologist never commented about it, but Claudia dreaded these appointments. After two or three years, she simply stopped going back.

Suggestions for Using Dilators Comfortably

If you have had radiation therapy or pelvic cancer surgery, and the instructions you were given about vaginal dilation are different from the ones in this book, follow your own doctor's advice. For most women, however, the program of dilator use described here can be helpful in reducing pain during sex related to pelvic muscle tension.

You should never have to force a dilator into your vagina. Using the dilator should not hurt, though you may notice slight discomfort at first.

Women often worry that using a dilator is a form of masturbation, for the purpose of sexual excitement and orgasm. Using a dilator is a treatment for pain with intercourse. Many women do not find the dilation sexually exciting. For those who do have sexual feelings with use of a dilator, they are quite normal and will not harm you.

Now you are ready to learn how to use your smallest dilator. Schedule time to practice with your dilator every other day. You should not spend more than ten or fifteen minutes each time you practice. If you use this schedule, you will practice often enough to make progress but still have time in between for any slight irritation of your vulva or vagina to clear up. Practicing for too long makes many women feel frustrated or anxious. Stretching out your practice sessions to once or twice a week also may lessen their effectiveness.

Choose a time when you feel relaxed, for example, after a bath or a shower. If the dilator feels cold to the touch, you can run warm water over it and dry it off. Smooth some water-based lubricant over the end of the smallest dilator and place the tip at the entrance of your vagina. Use a mirror to find your vaginal entrance if you wish. You can use the dilator lying on the bed, sitting up against some pillows or a headboard, or even lying in a warm bath.

Step 1: Squeeze your PC muscle, and then let it relax before gently sliding the dilator into your vagina. If you feel tension and the dilator does not slide easily, just slip it in a little way and hold it still. Tense the PC muscle again. You may feel the muscle push on the dilator as if to push it out of your vagina. Let the PC muscle relax and slip the dilator in a little farther. If you are not sure how your vagina angles back, wiggle the dilator gently and let the path of least resistance be your guide. You may need to tense and relax the PC muscle several times before the dilator slides in fully. When your muscles are relaxed, it should slide forward with only light pressure.

You will know the dilator is in fully when it will not move farther comfortably. The base of the dilator will be close to your vaginal entrance, but not inside. Take a moment to experience how the dilator feels inside of your vagina. Then remove it, sliding it gently out. You can wash the dilator off with a mild soap and water (but if you are using an electric vibrator as a dilator, remember that it should never be used around water!). Be sure to rinse all the soap off thoroughly so that residue will not remain to irritate your vagina the next time you use the dilator. If Step 1 was physically uncomfortable or made you feel tense, repeat it once or twice each practice session until you are more relaxed. If Step 1 was easy, you can go straight to Step 2.

Step 2:   Insert the lubricated, smallest dilator fully, but instead of removing it right away, hold it still in your vagina for several minutes. The goal is to hold the dilator in your vagina for seven to ten minutes without discomfort. Sometimes you will reach your goal the first time, but it also may take several tries, over several practice sessions. You can read or watch TV to help the time pass. You will probably have to hold the dilator in place with one hand because otherwise it tends to slip out of your vagina.

Step 3:   Insert the lubricated, smallest dilator. Hold it still for a moment and then try moving it around. Wiggle it gently from side to side. Slide it part of the way in and out of your vagina. Notice that you can feel the dilator move inside of your vagina without any pain or discomfort. Again, if this step is not completely comfortable the first time, repeat it over the next practice sessions until you feel you have mastered it.

Moving to a Larger Dilator: When you have completed Step 3 comfortably with the smallest dilator, you are ready to start over again with Step 1 on the next size of dilator. Do not be surprised if it is a little more difficult or uncomfortable to insert a larger dilator. You may need to practice Steps 1 to 3 with the new dilator for several practice sessions before you are able to relax fully. Soon the new size should become as comfortable as the smaller size was.

Each time you have completed Step 3 comfortably with a new size of dilator, you can go to Step 1 with the next size, until you can use your largest dilator comfortably. Do not be discouraged if a larger size is much more uncomfortable at first than the smaller sizes were. If you experience bleeding after dilator use or sharp pain from the dilator, however, consult your physician before going on.

Getting Help from Your Partner

If you currently have a sexual relationship, you may be wondering how using vaginal dilators will help you resume lovemaking. The first goal of using dilators is to learn that *you* are in control of your vagina. The next goal is to stay relaxed while your partner inserts a finger or dilator into your vagina.

Many women who have pain with vaginal penetration are able to enjoy having the outer part of their vulva caressed by a partner. If you can enjoy hand or oral caressing of your clitoris and vulvar area without pain, it is helpful to continue this type of lovemaking during the weeks you are practicing with your dilators. You and your partner can caress each other and even bring each other to orgasm through hand or oral sex, but you should avoid trying any penetration of your vagina.

When you feel ready, you can ask your partner to insert the smallest dilator into your vagina. This could be an experiment during a session of lovemaking, or perhaps you could have your partner join you at the end of one of your private practice times with the dilators. Of course the dilator should be lubricated. Your goal is to stay relaxed as you gradually transfer control from you to your partner. Again, you should go step by step:

Step 1: Have your partner put a hand over yours as you insert the smallest dilator. Remember to squeeze and relax your PC muscle just before you begin. Take the dilator out.

Step 2: Let your partner hold the dilator, but put your hand over your partner's to guide the insertion. Ask your partner to wait to begin until you signal you are ready.

Step 3: Let your partner put in the dilator solo, still following your instructions on when you are relaxed and ready. Your partner can practice holding the dilator gently in your vagina and moving it around.

After you feel relaxed with Step 3, you can go up a dilator size, returning to Step 1. Stay at least a size behind the one that you are using in your individual practice.

Another way to make the transition from dilators to intercourse is to have your partner begin to use a finger to caress the inside of your vagina during lovemaking. Choose a time when you are already feeling aroused by some kissing and caressing, so that your vagina is expanded and lubricated. Have your partner put some lubricant gel on a finger, and guide your partner either with your hand or in words, giving the signal that you are ready for your partner to slip a finger into your vagina. Again, you can use a Kegel to make sure your PC muscles are relaxed first. When caressing with one finger no longer causes discomfort, your partner can try gently putting two fingers inside of your vagina. When you feel comfortable with

your largest dilator and can enjoy caressing with two fingers in your vagina, you should be ready to try penile penetration.

Making a Transition to Penile-Vaginal Intercourse

I certainly do not mean to imply that intercourse with the man's penis
inside of the woman's vagina is the only enjoyable or normal way to have
sex. As you may have noticed, intercourse tends to be the most problematic sexual activity for women with genital pain. Some couples may never
have included vaginal penetration as part of lovemaking, and others can
give it up with few regrets. For heterosexual couples in America, however,
intercourse remains the most common and favored sexual practice and is
the goal that most of my patients choose.

Even when you have completed all the other steps, you should still
approach intercourse gradually. A first step is to be able to have penetration without discomfort. You will need your partner's patience and understanding because you are just going to try penetration, without going on
to the movement of intercourse. If you and your partner are comfortable
bringing each other to orgasm through hand caressing of the genital area
or through oral sex, you can agree to finish your lovemaking with
nonintercourse stimulation.

Your partner needs to have enough of an erection for penetration, lying still while you guide his penis into your vagina at your own pace. The
easiest position for this type of penetration is with the woman on top.
Your partner can lie on his back or sit up against some pillows or the
headboard of the bed. You can kneel facing him, with one knee on each
side of his body. Make sure to spread a gel lubricant on the head of his
penis and around the entrance of your vagina so that both surfaces are
slippery. Hold your partner's penis at the entrance of your vagina and do
a Kegel squeeze and release to make sure your PC muscle is relaxed. Slowly
sit down onto his penis. If the entrance to your vagina feels tight or tender at some point, stay at that depth of penetration and again squeeze and
release your PC muscle around your partner's penis. When you can feel
that your vagina is more relaxed, try to slide down a little more onto your
partner's penis. Penetration becomes a gradual process, with several Kegel
squeezes and releases before you slide down all the way. When you get
there, take a moment to experience how it feels to have the penis inside
of your vagina without moving around. Then slowly slide back up and off
of your partner's penis.

Some women feel tense when they are in the position above the man. They prefer to have their partner be on top, even though a woman has less control over penetration when she is on the bottom. If you find the woman-on-top position does not work well, by all means experiment with other positions that you think will work better. If you are on the bottom, you can hold your partner's penis with your hand to guide the angle of penetration. Ask him to prop himself on his hands so that his weight is not resting on you. Tell him when to gently push his penis into your vagina. Feel free to ask him to stop at any point so that you can use a Kegel squeeze to relax before he slides his penis farther inside.

Once penetration becomes fairly easy, you can experiment with the movements of intercourse. At first, it would be helpful if your partner would stay still and let you move your hips slowly and gently. Is there any angle or depth of penetration that still causes discomfort? Can you begin to feel pleasure as you feel your partner's penis inside of your vagina? Over several tries, your partner can become more active in moving during intercourse, and the two of you can experiment with different positions for penetration and movement.

After Intercourse Is Pain-Free

Once you and your partner can enjoy intercourse without pain, you may not need to use your dilators again. If you begin to feel a return of tension, however, or if you have some tightness with penetration, you may want to have more practice sessions with your dilators.

Intercourse Positions That Minimize Pain

Sex manuals and erotic stories have probably overemphasized the role of intercourse positions in enhancing sexual pleasure. Whole books and videos have been devoted to the idea that finding the right position for intercourse will transform a couple's sex life (see The Sexuality Library catalog in Resources under Products to Enhance Sex). Positions can make a difference, however, when a woman is having pain with intercourse.

As I mentioned while discussing dilators, a woman who is having pain and tightness with penetration may be able to stay more relaxed and in control if she is the partner on top and gently and gradually sits down onto her partner's erection while he stays still. Once penetration is complete, the couple can roll over into a different position if they prefer.

Some women who have pelvic cancer surgery or radiation are left with chronic tenderness at the top of the vagina that is set off by deep thrusting during intercourse. For them, it is best to avoid positions that involve deep penetration. Positions that are apt to be most painful include the woman lying on her back with her knees bent sharply up or with her feet on her partner's shoulders or the woman kneeling with her partner thrusting into her vagina from behind her. Instead, she may want to try being the partner on top or having intercourse lying on one side with her partner facing her or lying "like a spoon" behind her.

If a woman's vagina has become shallow or if she has tenderness deep inside, she may want to put some extra lubricant on her upper thighs and have intercourse with her thighs squeezed together. Her partner will get extra friction on his penis from rubbing against her upper thighs instead of penetrating deeply into her vagina. Unfortunately, however, many women have always held their thighs wide apart during lovemaking and have a hard time reaching orgasm with their thighs squeezed together. An alternative is for a woman to put lubricant on her hand and to circle the base of her partner's penis with her thumb and fingers. Then he will thrust partially against her hand and partially into her vagina, without reaching the deeper area that is painful.

Men Coping with Genital Pain

Genital pain in men is even more difficult to diagnose and treat than pain in women. A man who has pain may sometimes benefit from the pain-relieving qualities of an antidepressant. For men who have aching in their scrotum after cancer treatment, one of my urologist colleagues recommends rubbing a small amount of aspirin cream on the skin. You can also try the male version of Kegel exercises, squeezing the muscle that shuts off your urine flow and then letting it relax, practicing for several minutes a day aside from urination. As in women, chronic tension in the pelvic floor muscles can contribute to pain during sex. You may want to read some of the sections in this chapter that pertain to women on medications to alleviate genital pain, using lubricants to avoid friction on tender areas, and intercourse positions. Similar techniques may help your own situation.

Now we turn our attention from sexuality as an expression of pleasure and intimacy to sex with the purpose of conceiving a child. Part III of the book discusses how cancer treatments interfere with fertility and the options available to those who wish to become parents.

FERTILITY AND PREGNANCY: WHEN CANCER ADDS INSULT TO INJURY

15

Empty Arms: The Pain of Infertility

Infertility brings intense grief and anger to men and women who have never had a life-threatening illness. After experiencing cancer, to be infertile adds insult to injury. Because cancer becomes more common with age, most people have completed their families before the disease strikes. For survivors of childhood cancer, however, or for men or women who have cancer in their young adulthood, infertility is a frequent and painful issue.

Men or women who are infertile often feel defective or incomplete. Cancer survivors struggle already with feeling like damaged goods. Infertility is an added burden. Some men or women see infertility as a loss of their essential masculinity or femininity.

Infertility May Come as a Surprise

Infertility often comes as a surprise to cancer survivors. Many do not recall being warned at the time of their treatment that they were risking their fertility. Some were just not informed. Studies show that many present adults who had childhood cancer were not even told they had cancer, much less prepared for long-term side effects of treatment. Parents may have been aware of infertility as a future issue but hesitated to hurt their son or daughter more by revealing it.

Oncologists today give families more information and advocate honesty about cancer and its side effects, but infertility may still not be discussed in detail. Sometimes infertility is just mentioned as one of a list of negative effects of cancer treatment when a physician asks a patient to give "informed consent." At such a time of anxiety, few people can pro-cess all the frightening and complex information they are given.

Grieving over Lost Potential

The most profound loss is giving up the dream of having one's own, ge-netic child. Cancer survivors are often told by physicians, family, and well-meaning friends that they should be glad to be alive. Their pain at being infertile is dismissed as ingratitude. But many people see having a child as a very concrete way of defeating death and leaving a part of oneself for the future. Most men and women grow up assuming they will be parents one day. For a couple, that longed-for child was to be the blending of their individual strengths and the product of their love. Mental health profes-sionals who treat infertile couples often point out that it is difficult for them to grieve adequately or to get true understanding and support from family or friends because what has been lost is a potential, rather than an actual, child. The loss is no less real, however.

Infertility as a Barrier in New Relationships

Infertility is an issue in the marriage market. Cancer survivors already may worry that their health history will cause potential mates to reject them. Disclosing cancer treatment is a major hurdle in a dating relationship (see Chapter 28). It is even more difficult to discuss limits on fertility with a desirable mate. Even men or women who were already married when di-agnosed with cancer often fear that a spouse will leave after fertility is compromised—and infertility sometimes is a factor when younger couples break up after cancer treatment.

Infertility Brings Tough Choices

Cancer survivors who face infertility must make difficult choices with little available guidance from experts. The chance of living a normal life span remains uncertain for a number of years after cancer treatment. How soon after cancer should you try for a pregnancy? Will the cancer return? Are you at increased risk for a new malignancy later in your life or for other long-term health problems related to radiation therapy or chemotherapy?

You do not have the luxury of waiting many years before you try to conceive. Biological clocks do not stop ticking. For women, some chemotherapies leave only a short window of fertility before a premature menopause. Cancer treatment can also affect the ability to carry a healthy pregnancy. Cancer survivors may worry about the risk of birth defects in their children or the chance that offspring will themselves be at high risk to develop cancer.

Infertility treatment is expensive and often not covered by insurance policies. Men or women who have survived cancer may already have suffered financially from medical bills, from loss of salary, or their disease interfering with advancement at work. Adoption has also become increasingly expensive and complex. How should you invest your hopes, money, and effort? Choosing to pursue private adoption or to have high-technology treatments like in vitro fertilization often means prioritizing and giving up other goals for the family. For some couples, these options are simply not affordable under any circumstances. Whatever avenue you choose, you must cope not only with the uncertainty of your disease, but also with the lack of control you ultimately have over becoming a parent.

Cheryl had surgery and chemotherapy for a germ-cell tumor of one ovary at age 24. She was already engaged to marry when her cancer was diagnosed. Three years later, she and her husband decided to try for a pregnancy. Cheryl knew that her remaining ovary was functioning well, but she found the eight months it took to get pregnant nerve-racking. She took her temperature monthly and made sure to have sex every day during the crucial week. Having intercourse became a chore that had to be done before breakfast or at midnight when she just wanted to go to sleep. Sometimes her husband had trouble getting erections, and she felt so angry at him that she wanted to scream.

Ultimately, Cheryl did become pregnant, but her anxiety did not end with the positive test. Every day she imagined that her baby would be born with some abnormality or that she would miscarry. Her husband had a hard time being sympathetic to her worries, but ultrasounds helped reassure her that the baby was developing normally. Toward the end of her pregnancy, she had premature contractions. She spent a night in the hospital and was then on bed rest. Because the baby was breech, Cheryl ended up with a C-section. As soon as she heard the baby cry, she asked if she had all her fingers and toes. Although the baby was healthy, Cheryl feels tense about having a daughter, worrying about her child's future risk of cancer. On the other hand, she is very grateful to have a baby and feels more like a normal person than she has since her cancer was diagnosed.

Choosing to Live without Children

Not everyone has a dream of being a parent. Children bring a good deal of stress as well as joy. Many men and women value the freedom to pursue absorbing careers or hobbies. Perhaps going through your experience with cancer also changed your priorities or your readiness to take on the long-term responsibility of parenthood. Although our society still gives a basic message that having children is a very high priority, we have many more nontraditional models of adult life as well.

Even if you began your adult life expecting to be a parent eventually, going through cancer treatment and facing infertility may have changed your perspective. Some men and women fight for fertility for years, going through a series of unsuccessful infertility treatments before they feel ready to let go and grieve for their loss. Sometimes one partner in a couple is ready to give up, while the other still wants to pursue infertility treatment or adoption. If you are having trouble accepting infertility, some counseling with a mental health professional familiar with the issues may be helpful.

Finding Emotional Support

Anyone who is coping with infertility should be aware of the organization Resolve, a national information clearinghouse that also sponsors local chapters and support groups (see Resources under Information Networks). You may also find other support groups in your community for people facing infertility. It can be very helpful to share your experiences with others and to get some empathy. Mental health professionals familiar with infertility issues also offer individual and couple counseling. To find such a specialist, try contacting infertility clinics in your area.

Besides coping with your sadness about infertility, you may also be able to take practical steps to fulfill your dream of having a child. The next chapter suggests ways to find the professional help you may need to overcome infertility after cancer treatment.

16

Maybe a Baby? Researching Your Options

Some men and women are lucky enough to be fertile after cancer treatment and to conceive without difficulty when they are ready. Many men and women need special treatment if they are to have a chance at conception, however. When couples have no known risk for infertility, they are usually advised to have intercourse regularly for a year without using birth control before seeking medical help. You may want to be more proactive, however, and consult an infertility specialist when you are ready to try for a pregnancy or after a shorter period of failing to conceive.

Finding the Right Infertility Specialist

Because treatment for infertility is expensive and often is not covered by insurance, your options may unfortunately be limited by finances. (But be sure to check with your health insurance carrier so you know what to expect.) If you are going to invest your money and physical and emotional effort into infertility treatment, go for the best care you can afford. Many gynecologists or urologists who provide infertility treatment have not had extra training beyond their residencies. Some may be excellent, but your best strategy is to find a physician with specialty credentials in infertility.

Look for a gynecologist who is also a board-certified reproductive endocrinologist. Finding a urologist with special training in male infertility is more difficult. A few urologists around the country have had a year or two of fellowship training in infertility after they finished their residency in urology. If you are going to an infertility clinic, choose a program that offers expertise in both female and male infertility. If you do not live near a large city, it may be worth your while to travel to the nearest urban center with a successful infertility clinic. You should also ask if your infertility specialists have had experience with treating cancer survivors. More information about finding an infertility specialist can be obtained by contacting the American Society for Reproductive Medicine (see Resources under Information Networks).

The Society for Assisted Reproductive Technology (SART) keeps statistics on the success rates of infertility clinics that use such high-technology procedures as in vitro fertilization (IVF). Because of a number of scandals about unscrupulous advertising by infertility clinics and the threat of government regulation, almost all clinics participate in the SART registry. You can get reports on infertility clinics in your region by contacting SART through the American Society for Reproductive Medicine. Reports are kept separately for standard IVF, gamete intrafallopian transfer (GIFT), zygote intrafallopian transfer (ZIFT), and transfer of frozen embryos. Information on egg donation is also gathered. Be an informed and aware consumer.

Tests That Measure a Man's Fertility

How can a man know if he is fertile after cancer treatment? All of the tests are designed to measure whether his testicles are producing enough healthy sperm cells.

The Semen Analysis

If a man can ejaculate semen, he can have a test called semen analysis. A man should not ejaculate through partner sex or masturbation for two to three days before giving a semen sample. Then he brings the semen to a special laboratory as soon as possible after ejaculation. Most labs prefer to have the man masturbate into a collection cup in a private room right on the premises, but an alternative is to collect semen at home, keeping it at body temperature (for example, by putting the container in a pants or shirt pocket) and getting it to the lab within an hour. For men who cannot ejaculate outside of intercourse, for example, because of a religious issue, a special silicone collection condom can be provided. Regular latex condoms damage the sample. The semen is examined with a microscope and often with automated testing machines. Ask if the laboratory provides computerized sperm counts and is certified by the appropriate national organization.

Several factors are important in male fertility:

- The *semen volume* is the amount of liquid ejaculated. A normal quantity would be 1.5 to 5.0 milliliters (ml). Five milliliters equals a teaspoon.
- The *sperm count* is the number of sperm cells seen in a certain amount of fluid. Normal would be more than 20 million in each milliliter of liquid.
- The *motility* is the percentage of sperm cells actively swimming in the liquid. Normally more than 50 percent of sperm are motile.
- The *percent normal forms* is the percent of sperm cells that have a normally shaped head. It should be more than 30 percent.

Sperm cells should not be sticking to each other. The seminal fluid should not contain an unusual number of white or red blood cells. The viscosity (texture and thickness) of the semen should be right. A semen analysis is often repeated on two or three occasions to make sure all the values are stable.

Hormone Tests

For men who do not ejaculate semen or who have very low sperm counts, another common test is to analyze a blood sample for follicle-stimulating hormone (FSH), which is produced by the pituitary gland and regulates sperm cell production in the testicles. If all is normal, FSH levels vary between 2 and 10 international units in each liter (IU/l) of blood. When the testicles have been damaged, FSH levels rise. If a man's FSH level is double or triple the normal range, he may be permanently unable to produce sperm cells.

Testicular Biopsies

A sample of tissue from the testicle can also be removed in a minor surgery called a *testicular biopsy* and examined to see if some sperm production is under way. With recent advances in treating severe male infertility, even men with very high FSH levels have been found to produce some sperm cells in their testicles that can be harvested during a biopsy and used for assisted reproduction.

Tests That Measure a Woman's Fertility

The most common fertility question for a woman after cancer treatment is whether she is *ovulating* (producing ripe eggs) normally. A useful concept in understanding infertility after cancer is *ovarian reserve* (the ovaries' remaining capacity to produce ripe eggs). A woman is born with all the eggs she will ever have. Every woman experiences some decline in her fertility starting in her early thirties, because the number and quality of her eggs decrease. Some get used up each month, and others are exposed to environmental damage. A young woman given chemotherapy drugs or radiation may end up with little ovarian reserve, similar to a woman of older age.

Hormone Tests

If a woman is having regular menstrual cycles (between twenty-one and thirty-five days long) and is not having hot flashes, chances are that she is ovulating. But how well are her ovaries functioning? Ovarian reserve can be estimated by the results of a blood test for FSH. If a woman is menstruating, the blood is sampled on the second or third day of her cycle. Each laboratory has different values for FSH, but typically a normal level at this point in the cycle would be under 10 IU/l. A woman in permanent menopause has an FSH greater than 40 IU/l.

The FSH level for women whose ovarian reserve is decreased falls in the middle. If FSH is above 18 IU/l, even strong fertility drugs may not stimulate the ovaries to ripen enough eggs for procedures such as in vitro fertilization. If FSH is over 25 IU/l, women may be advised to consider using eggs from a donor, rather than trying infertility treatment to stimulate their own ovaries. Age also is a factor, however, and a very young woman with a somewhat increased FSH level after cancer treatment may still have a chance for pregnancy. Blood tests for luteinizing hormone (LH), progesterone, or estrogen can also be helpful indicators of fertility.

Monitoring Ovulation

Ovulation can also be monitored directly. Women can use a special thermometer to take their temperature each morning on waking. A monthly chart of temperature changes can give clues about whether ovulation is taking place. Pharmacies now sell special ovulation prediction kits without a prescription that women can use around the middle of their menstrual cycle to test their urine. The test measures a hormone surge that signals ovulation. These kits are expensive, however, and usually are used when a woman is trying to get pregnant and wants to make sure to have intercourse at the right time of the month. During infertility treatment, ovulation is often monitored by getting ultrasound pictures of the ovary that can show follicles containing ripening eggs.

Endometrial Biopsies

An *endometrial biopsy* consists of taking a small sample of the uterine lining two or three days before the expected menstrual period to make sure the lining has developed properly. This test measures whether the uterus would be receptive to an embryo, allowing it to implant and grow. Endometrial biopsies are uncomfortable because the physician must put a small tube through the cervix to get the sample tissue, but they are routinely done in the doctor's office.

Testing the Fallopian Tubes and Uterus

Although cancer treatment rarely damages the uterus or fallopian tubes, the health of these organs is crucial to a woman's fertility. By means of a *hysterosalpingogram* (a special X ray that records images of the uterus and fallopian tubes made possible by a dye injected through the cervix), abnormalities in the uterine cavity or tubes can be seen. A newer way to view the inside of the uterus is *office hysteroscopy* (a small, flexible telescope is passed through the cervix). Problems in the pelvis can also be diagnosed by a *laparoscopy* (a minor surgery in which a small incision is created in the area of the navel to allow a lighted telescope to see into the pelvis). During laparoscopy, scar tissue or endometriosis blocking the tubes or ovaries can be treated with cautery or laser.

The Postcoital Test

The postcoital test evaluates the quality of the cervical mucus, which should become thinner and easier for sperm to penetrate at the time of a woman's ovulation. The couple is asked to have intercourse, and then the woman's cervical mucus is examined within the next several hours to see if it is the right consistency and if live sperm cells are present.

Once you know the results of your infertility evaluation, you can make a more informed choice among the different treatment options that are open to you. The rest of the chapters in this section explain some of those alternatives.

17

Sperm Manufacture: When Cancer Treatment Shuts Down the Line

Cancer treatment commonly causes male infertility by damaging sperm cell production. To understand why, you need a basic knowledge of how sperm cells ripen. Sperm cells are produced by a man's testicles beginning at puberty. During the rest of his life, even into old age, a man will continue to make new sperm cells. Sperm cells are produced by special stem cells that are present from birth. Once the stem cell produces an unripe sperm cell, however, the offshoot cell goes through several stages before it becomes mature seventy-four days later. During this time, the ripening sperm cell divides rapidly, more rapidly than other cells. When a cell is in the midst of dividing, its genetic material is fragile. Cancer cells also divide much more often than most normal cells. Indeed, this is the reason that radiation and chemotherapy can kill cancer cells without killing the patient. Unfortunately, the rapidly dividing sperm cells are also vulnerable to damage.

Radiation Therapy and Sperm Cells

To treat a tumor, a typical dose of radiation therapy would be 2500 to 7500 *rad* (the unit of measurement for radiation) aimed directly at the cancer. Unfortunately, it only takes 600 rad to the testicles to destroy a man's fertility permanently by killing off all the stem cells.

The testicles are occasionally the *direct* target of radiation, for example, in treating some leukemias or testicular cancers (seminoma). But they are in danger from indirect radiation also. Specially shaped sheets of lead can shield the testicles to reduce their exposure to radiation given to the pelvis to treat, for example, cancer of the prostate. And, the farther away the radiation target is from the testicles, the lower the dose they receive. However, radiation tends to scatter inside the body, bouncing off organs and lymph nodes and getting redirected, like a bullet ricocheting. Thus, the testicles may get some radiation even if the field is not nearby.

Because ripening sperm cells are more sensitive than the stem cells, a dose of radiation below 600 rad to the testicles will slow down or stop sperm cell production. However, sperm counts can recover within a few months to several years—the higher the dose, the longer the time to recover.

Age also plays a part in radiation damage: The testicles of boys who have not reached puberty are more resistant to radiation than those of an adult—it takes a higher dose to do the same amount of damage as in an adult.

Chemotherapy and Sperm Cells

The impact of chemotherapy drugs on sperm production in men is similar in many ways to the effects of radiation. Chemotherapy damages the rapidly dividing, ripening sperm cells. If damage is severe, the stem cells die as well. The higher the total dose of a damaging chemotherapy drug, the more slowly sperm cell production recovers, or the more likely it is to stop permanently. In fact, the worst damage to fertility occurs when men are treated with a combination of radiation therapy to the abdomen or pelvis and chemotherapy that includes drugs damaging to fertility.

Some chemotherapy drugs seem to have little impact on sperm cell production. The effects of others are not yet fully understood. One class of drug known to damage fertility are the alkylating chemotherapies. Alkylating drugs include cyclophosphamide (Cytoxan), chlorambucil, busulfan, procarbazine, nitrosoureas, nitrogen mustard, and l-phenylalanine mustard. Some of these drugs are included in chemotherapy commonly given for Hodgkin's disease or other lymphomas.

Recently, efforts have been made to change the treatments for Hodgkin's disease to drug combinations that are less damaging to fertility. Men treated for testicular cancer usually do not receive alkylating drugs. After combination chemotherapy for testicular cancer that includes VP-16, cis-platinum, or bleomycin, about half of men recover normal sperm counts.

Boys who have not reached puberty may be less likely to have permanent damage to their fertility than are teenagers or adults. Recovery of sperm production after chemotherapy in adult men is slow, usually occurring one to four years after the end of treatment. If recovery has not taken place by four years, it is unlikely, however. Men over age 40 are less likely to recover fertility.

Can Sperm Cells Be Protected?

Because the testicles appear to resist damage before puberty, researchers thought that inactivating the testicles might protect sperm production during cancer treatment. Several different hormone treatments have been used to turn off sperm cell production, but none has proven successful in protecting men's fertility. Once sperm cell production is damaged, there is no way to repair it, although modern infertility treatments can sometimes create a pregnancy with only a few sperm cells (see Chapter 18). A better option is preserving some healthy sperm cells before cancer treatment begins.

The Icemen Cometh: Sperm Banking before Cancer Treatment

Because it is known that some cancer treatments damage fertility, men should be offered the option to bank sperm before pelvic surgery, radiation therapy, or chemotherapy. Many men are not offered sperm banking because their physicians lack knowledge about infertility and its treatment or think the issue is not important. A number of young men who could bank sperm decide not to because they believe they will escape infertility or because they have a hard time imagining that they will one day want children. Unfortunately, research has shown that many of these men regret their decision later in life.

Vinnie was only 15 when his Hodgkin's disease was diagnosed. His treatment included both radiation therapy and chemotherapy. He recalls the oncologist saying something about fertility and banking sperm to him and his parents before beginning cancer treatment. "I think he downplayed it, though. He said it was expensive, and he wasn't sure if the stuff would still be good by the time I was married and wanted kids. I remember my mother asking if it would delay my treatment and being really upset at the idea of waiting a couple of extra weeks. Then the doctor kind of mumbled something about collecting semen by masturbation, and my mother blushed bright red. At the time, I used to play with myself daily, but I sure wasn't going to admit that to my mom and dad! I think I told my parents not to worry, that I could always adopt."

Now Vinnie is 26 and engaged. He had a semen analysis, and no live sperm were found. He and his fiancée have discussed both adoption and conceiving a child through donor insemination. Vinnie cannot get over feeling like he is cheating her, although she has been loving and supportive. Sometimes he looks back with anger, feeling that his doctor could have done a better job of explaining the importance of sperm banking. "He should have thought about how I would feel years later. At 15, I sure couldn't imagine it. I was too busy worrying about having to drop out of basketball!"

How Does Sperm Banking Work?

In most large cities, a sperm bank is available. Some cancer centers or large hospitals have their own sperm banks. If a man does not live near a sperm bank, a laboratory can collect and freeze semen for shipping to a storage bank. Then, when a couple is ready to try for a pregnancy, the semen can be shipped to them.

Normally, two weeks are allowed to collect enough semen samples for banking, but men who need to start cancer treatment can often collect a useful amount of semen within a few days. Men are asked not to ejaculate by any means for twenty-four to forty-eight hours before each sample of semen is collected. A man will need to give three to six samples to store enough semen to give him and his partner the best chance of conception later on. The number of samples recommended will be higher if the semen is not high in quality.

The sample is collected through masturbation in a private room at the laboratory. Most laboratories allow a man to bring his partner with him to help with manual stimulation. Even though special collection condoms made of silicone can be used in intercourse to obtain a sample of semen, this collection method is not advised for sperm banking because it increases the risk of contaminating the semen with bacteria. For the same reason, oral sex is not a good method of semen collection.

The semen is collected on site because sperm cells die easily, especially if the semen is allowed to cool gradually. The semen is flash-frozen in liquid nitrogen as soon as possible after ejaculation to maximize its quality. Freezing and thawing semen always does some damage, reducing the number of live sperm cells in the sample or making them less active. Once the semen is frozen, however, it can be stored for up to fifty years without deteriorating over time. Typically, the sperm bank charges the man an annual storage fee.

You may be told that you are not a good candidate for sperm banking. Many men with cancer start out with poor fertility, even before active treatment. Most of these men do not have a long history of infertility; but once the cancer becomes active, fevers, physical stress, and sometimes hormones produced by the tumor can interfere with sperm production.

About three-quarters of men with testicular cancer have reduced sperm counts and motility soon after diagnosis. Men with testicular cancer have typically had recent surgery to remove one testicle when they are sent for sperm banking. The anesthesia during surgery can temporarily decrease sperm cell ripening. A minority of men with testicular cancer also start out with lifelong infertility because of abnormalities in both testicles. Semen quality is also commonly affected in men with lymphoma or Hodgkin's disease. A recent study of sixty-two young men with cancer who banked sperm at The Cleveland Clinic Foundation showed that sperm count and motility were often abnormal before freezing. The type of cancer did not affect the likelihood of poor semen quality. The process of freezing and thawing the semen did not have any worse impact on these samples than it did for healthy men, however.

Usually, men are advised not to bank sperm if the count or motility is below normal. For men with cancer, however, banking may be worthwhile even when semen quality is not very good. Not only may the frozen semen be a man's only chance to father a genetic child, but new techniques of infertility treatment make each sperm cell precious, as we will see in the next chapter. And there has not been any increased risk of birth defects observed in babies conceived with frozen semen.

Stem Cell Banking?

In the next several years, it may become possible to harvest some stem cells from the testicles, freeze them, and return them to a man after his cancer treatment. Testicular stem cell transplants have already been successful in animal research, but have not yet been tried in humans.

Fortunately, as we will see in the next chapter, new treatments can help men father children even when sperm counts and motility are very low. The trick is to help nature by getting the sperm and the egg together.

18

Special Delivery: Getting the Sperm to the Egg

If a man has some healthy sperm cells available, infertility treatment after cancer may require some special ways of getting the sperm and egg to meet.

Dealing with Orgasm Problems

As we saw in Chapter 12, having dry orgasms does not ruin a man's sex life. It does make conception difficult, however. One strategy is to modify cancer treatment so that dry orgasm is less common as a side effect.

Preventing Dry Orgasm in Men with Testicular Cancer

Dry orgasm is most often a barrier to fertility in men treated with retroperitoneal node dissection surgery for nonseminomatous tumors of the testicle (a fast-growing type of testicular cancer). The goal of this surgery is to decide whether a man needs chemotherapy. Modern chemotherapy drugs are so successful in treating testicular cancer, however, that cancer specialists have felt comfortable modifying the criteria for node dissection.

For men with small tumors confined to the testicle itself (Stage I cancer), the node dissection surgery can sometimes be skipped. Treatment stops with surgery to remove the testicle and its cord. No radiation therapy or chemotherapy is given and most men will have good fertility. Careful cancer surveillance is crucial to this approach, however. Around 30 percent of men with early stage nonseminomas will eventually develop metastases. They need immediate treatment, or their life will be in danger. Surveillance is expensive because sophisticated medical tests must be repeated every several months. Young men with testicular cancer are also not always faithful in keeping their follow-up appointments, leading to a slightly higher death rate than expected in surveillance programs. For the man who is very conscientious about his health, however, and is concerned about preserving his fertility, surveillance may be an option.

Another way to avoid dry orgasm is to have a modified retroperitoneal nerve dissection, in which some of the nerves that control emission are spared by limiting the extent of surgery. A higher percentage of men (50 percent to 90 percent, depending on the technique used) continue to ejaculate normally after nerve-sparing node dissections. Another group of men has a temporary failure to ejaculate semen but recovers over the next one to three years. Many centers offer nerve-sparing surgery, but some urologists worry that limiting the node dissection makes it a less effective tool in cancer treatment.

Retrieving Sperm Cells in Men with Dry Orgasm

Even if a man does not ejaculate semen after his cancer treatment, it is often possible to retrieve his live sperm cells.

• Retrieving Sperm Cells from the Testicle. After surgery removing the prostate and seminal vesicles, such as radical prostatectomy or radical cystectomy, semen is no longer produced. Nevertheless, an infertility specialist can extract sperm cells from the tiny tubes where they ripen at the top of the testicles (epididymis) or even from a slice of tissue removed surgically from the testicle. These techniques involve outpatient surgery and should be done by an expert. If the *vasa deferentia* (tubes connecting the epididymis and seminal vesicles) are still in place, some urologists use a needle to obtain fluid containing sperm cells directly from one of them. Because all these procedures create scar tissue, they can only be tried a limited number of times. Luckily, most men who have radical pelvic surgery are past the age when they wish to father children.

• Medication That Restores Emission. Infertility can also be treated after operations that damage the nerves involved in emission of semen (see Chapter 12), including retroperitoneal lymph node dissection or some operations for cancer of the colon. Medication can sometimes stimulate the remaining nerves around the prostate and seminal vesicles. If the medication works, the glands contract, the internal valve at the bladder entrance closes, and semen spurts out of the penis at orgasm. The medication used most often in the United States is ephedrine sulfate. In Europe, imipramine (Tofranil) has also been used. These medications do not work for everyone, and they lose their effectiveness temporarily after a few doses. To maximize its usefulness, ephedrine sulfate is usually prescribed only for the week surrounding the wife's midcycle (the fertile period that typically starts twelve to fourteen days after the first day of her menstrual bleeding), and the couple is instructed to have intercourse daily during that period.

• Retrieving Sperm Cells from Urine. Sometimes medication does not produce normal ejaculation of semen but does get the prostate and seminal vesicles working again. The internal valve does not shut, however, and semen shoots backward into the bladder (retrograde ejaculation). To diagnose retrograde ejaculation, a man is asked to urinate right after he has an orgasm. The urine is tested for a chemical called *fructose* that is present in semen. Urine can also be examined under a microscope to see if sperm cells are present.

If a man has retrograde ejaculation, live sperm cells can sometimes be recovered from his urine. The man is given medication to make his urine less acid, avoiding damage to fragile sperm cells. He then has an orgasm through masturbation or use of a vibrator at the laboratory that will process his semen. Immediately after orgasm, his urine is collected through urination or catheterization, and the sperm cells are separated out. They are put into a special nutrient solution and used in infertility treatment.

• Stimulating Ejaculation with Electricity. If medication does not work, a technique called *electroejaculation* may also be used: A small probe placed in a man's anus produces an electrical pulse that stimulates ejaculation of semen. The semen is collected and used in infertility treatment. Currently, only a few centers around the United States offer electroejaculation. It must be performed under general anesthesia, or it would be very painful. For men whose spines have been damaged by cancer or its treatment and who have no sensation in the pelvic area, electroejaculation can be done without anesthesia.

Electroejaculation does not create scarring and so can be repeated on a number of occasions. It is less expensive than having surgery to extract sperm cells and sometimes yields better quality semen that can be used without resorting to in vitro fertilization, as we will see in a moment.

Inability to Reach Orgasm

A few men who want to father children may be unable to reach orgasm at all after cancer treatment. Several of the techniques in the preceding discussion can be used to retrieve their sperm, including extracting sperm by surgery or with a needle and electroejaculation. In addition, some infertility specialists have industrial-strength vibrators that can mechanically stimulate men to ejaculate even after spinal cord damage.

Making Every Sperm Count: Treatments That Bypass Low Sperm Counts or Low Motility

Men who recover some sperm production after chemotherapy or pelvic radiotherapy often have low counts or low motility. Similar problems occur when semen is banked and thawed. Sperm yield is even more limited from the just-described techniques for men who do not ejaculate normally. Until the past few years, men who had low sperm counts or low motility had little chance of fathering a child. The treatment of severe male infertility has recently taken a giant step, however.

Intrauterine Insemination

If sperm count and motility are only mildly decreased, semen can be used for intrauterine insemination (IUI), in which sperm cells are placed directly into a woman's uterus, using a small tube or syringe slipped through her cervix. The sperm cells are washed in a special procedure to separate them from the seminal fluid, eliminating chemicals that would cause the uterus to contract painfully. The IUI is done in a doctor's office without any anesthesia and is usually only momentarily uncomfortable. If the woman does not have optimal menstrual cycles, she may be given special hormones to stimulate her ovulation and increase the chances of pregnancy.

In Vitro Fertilization with Sperm Injection

In vitro fertilization (IVF) has been around for almost twenty years and involves giving a woman special hormones to stimulate her ovaries to ripen multiple eggs. The eggs are harvested by using an ultrasound-guided needle passed through the woman's upper vagina. Sperm cells are mixed with each egg in the laboratory. Eggs that are fertilized become embryos that can be transferred into the woman's uterus or frozen for future use.

When sperm counts or motility are very poor, IVF is not very successful. Now, however, a growing number of infertility centers use a new, high-tech treatment called in vitro fertilization with intracytoplasmic sperm injection (IVF-ICSI). The embryologist uses micromanipulation techniques to bring the sperm and egg together—under a microscope, a robotic machine injects one sperm cell directly into each egg. The first babies were born from IVF-ICSI in 1992, and success rates from IVF-ICSI now are equal to or better than those from conventional IVF for female infertility (see Chapter 19). Babies have been born when the father could only provide a few sperm cells, rather than the millions usually required. A drawback is that the woman bears the burden of discomfort and medical risks in IVF-ICSI, despite the fact that the man has the problem. She is also the major factor in its success. Pregnancy rates from ICSI are limited mainly by factors such as the woman's age and health, and not by the quality of the man's sperm. Not all IVF clinics offer ICSI, and it takes the embryologist a good deal of practice to learn to do the procedure successfully.

Whether IVF is used with or without ICSI, drawbacks include its expense, which can run between $5,000 and $10,000 for each cycle, and its limited success rates. As I was writing this book, the SART success rates for IVF for the United States and Canada had just been published for the year 1994. Overall, 33,700 cycles of IVF were performed that year. In an average of 20.7 percent of egg-retrieval procedures (i.e., at least one egg was harvested), a live birth resulted. Success rates of IVF-ICSI were not available separately, but an excellent clinic in 1996 can hit 30 percent to 40 percent live births per retrieval procedure when the woman is under age 35 and has normal fertility. IVF also produces a high rate of twin pregnancies. Only about 60 to 66 percent of IVF pregnancies are singletons. Most of the rest are twins, but triplets or more can also occur. Although some infertile couples rejoice in having "two for one," twin pregnancies increase the risk of miscarriage, prematurity, and other pregnancy complications. Rates of multiple births can be reduced by restricting the number of embryos placed into the mother's uterus. Responsible clinics usually limit the number of embryos to three, unless special circumstances suggest that replacing more embryos would increase the chances of a pregnancy.

Lee's testicular cancer was diagnosed when he was just 19 and a sophomore in college. He had a steady girlfriend but was far from thinking about having children. Before Lee had surgery to remove his lymph nodes, the surgeon warned him that he would probably have dry orgasms afterward. Techniques to spare the nerves were not yet in wide use when Lee's cancer was treated. Although Lee tried to bank sperm, he was told that his sperm counts and motility were too low to allow freezing to be useful. Again, the use of in vitro fertilization had not been widely popularized as a treatment for male infertility in those years, and sperm injection was not even dreamed of.

By the time Lee was 29 and married for two years, his infertility was the most painful issue in his life. Lee consulted a urologist who specialized in male infertility. Because Lee had dry orgasms, his urine was tested for sperm cells after ejaculation. None was found. Lee tried ephedrine. Although no semen appeared at orgasm, he did begin to have some sperm cells in his urine after using the medication. Lee and his wife went through six cycles in which sperm cells were gathered from his urine and used in intrauterine insemination. Although some live sperm were seen each time, Lee's wife did not become pregnant. They began to discuss living without children when Lee's urologist called to tell him that ICSI was being performed on a research basis at the center.

Lee and his wife were very lucky that their insurance covered three cycles of IVF. On the first cycle, Lee's wife produced sixteen eggs. Eight were fertilized through ICSI, and three embryos were transferred back into her uterus. The rest were frozen for a future transfer. Lee's wife became pregnant with twins. Although they were born somewhat prematurely, both were healthy. The couple plans to wait two or three years and then thaw their remaining embryos and try for a third child.

19

Women's Fertility: A Nonrenewable Resource

Women's fertility is especially vulnerable because it is nonrenewable. A woman is born with all the eggs she will ever have. She does not have cells that correspond to the stem cells that produce sperm cells in men. A uterus is also indispensable for having a baby; and if a woman has a hysterectomy, she has no options for reproducing, unless she involves another woman to carry her child (see Chapter 22). Let us review how a woman's reproductive system works.

Women's Reproductive Systems: What You Forgot from Health Class

Figure 19.1 gives a visual guide to a woman's reproductive system.

How Eggs Ripen

Each month after a woman reaches full maturity, as many as fifty eggs begin to ripen in one of her two ovaries. Each ripening egg, an *oocyte*, is surrounded by a nest of cells, a *follicle*. Typically, only one egg reaches full maturity each month. When the egg is ripe, the swollen follicle is filled with fluid and looks like a bubble about an inch in diameter on the surface of the ovary.

The cells in the follicle divide rapidly during the ripening process, making them especially vulnerable to damage by cancer treatments such

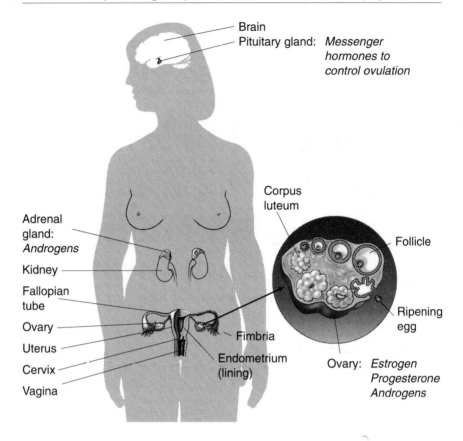

Brain
Pituitary gland: *Messenger hormones to control ovulation*

Corpus luteum

Adrenal gland: *Androgens*

Kidney

Fallopian tube

Ovary

Uterus

Cervix

Vagina

Fimbria

Endometrium (lining)

Follicle

Ripening egg

Ovary: *Estrogen Progesterone Androgens*

Figure 19.1   The woman's internal reproductive system

as radiation therapy and chemotherapy. The oocyte itself is not as fragile. An oocyte cannot ripen, however, if its follicle has been damaged.

The Egg's Journey

At ovulation, the follicle bursts open, and the ripe egg is swept into the fallopian tube by the fringelike *fimbria* that form the end of the tube. The follicle continues to produce hormones for the next couple of weeks. The ripe egg takes about two days to travel down the tube. It is only during these two days that the sperm cells can meet and fertilize the egg.

A woman's fertile days are usually around days 14 to 16 after the first bleeding of her menstrual period, but few women have perfectly regular menstrual cycles. In fact, from the first day of bleeding in one cycle to the first day of the next, a normal cycle can be anywhere from twenty-one to thirty-five days long. If a woman does not become pregnant (i.e., if the egg is not fertilized), the follicle stops producing hormones, and the lining of the uterus dissolves. The blood and tissue that formed the lining pass through her cervix as her menstrual flow.

After Fertilization

The fertilized egg, or *embryo*, continues the journey into the uterus, where it implants in the thick lining and the placenta begins to develop. In the ninth week after fertilization, the embryo is referred to as a *fetus*.

During the forty weeks of pregnancy, the single fertilized egg cell rapidly develops into a human infant. Because the fetus grows so rapidly and in such complex ways, birth defects can be caused if a woman is exposed to radiation therapy or chemotherapy during pregnancy. The fetus is especially fragile during the first trimester (thirteen weeks, or three months) of the pregnancy, when its basic structures are forming.

Cancer Treatments That Cause Infertility in Women

Surgery That Removes Crucial Parts

Removing both ovaries in surgery (bilateral oophorectomy) prevents conception because the woman no longer has any eggs. Women with one healthy ovary can usually get pregnant, however. Young women who lose one ovary to ovarian cancer have been able to preserve their fertility and have a child. Of course, any operation that removes the uterus (hysterectomy) prevents pregnancy because the fetus has no place to grow.

Less drastic operations in the pelvis can also occasionally damage a woman's fertility. Even if her uterus and ovaries remain untouched, scarring after surgery can narrow or block her fallopian tubes, interfering with the passage of the egg. Scar tissue can also sometimes displace or cover the ovaries themselves. Scarring can be diagnosed and sometimes removed in a minor surgical procedure called a laparoscopy (see Chapter 16).

Radiation Therapy and Women's Fertility

Radiation therapy can easily damage a woman's ovaries. Radiation damages the follicles and, at high doses, the oocytes themselves. The higher the dose of radiation, the more likely it is that infertility will be permanent. Doses between 600 and 1,000 rad (the units that measure radiation dose) to the ovary usually cause menopause. Lesser doses can temporarily halt menstruation but allow the possibility for fertility to recover.

The ovaries usually receive some damage if radiation is given to the lower spine, abdomen, or pelvis. The closer the target area of radiation is to the ovaries, the higher the radiation dose the ovaries receive. The ovaries can be shielded from a radiation source outside the body by covering the pelvic area with a lead apron. Still, the ovaries are hit by radiation that scatters when it is directed at other internal organs. When a source of radiation is placed temporarily inside the vagina (e.g., to treat cervical cancer), the ovaries also are bombarded with radiation.

In young women with Hodgkin's disease, an operation called oophoropexy is sometimes used to move the ovaries to an area behind the uterus. Then when radiation therapy is given to the shoulders and abdomen, the ovaries are less exposed to damage. Fertility is preserved in about half of women who have this protective surgery. Similar success in preserving the ovaries has been reported when they are moved outward to the sides of the pelvis in women who have hysterectomies for cancer of the cervix and then need radiation therapy. These women would not be able to carry a pregnancy, of course, because they have no uterus; but they would continue to produce estrogen instead of becoming menopausal. They might also be able to have eggs harvested for in vitro fertilization (IVF), followed by implantation in another woman's uterus (see Chapter 22).

When radiation therapy is used for cancers in childhood, the ovaries are less sensitive to damage. However, if a girl received a dose of radiation strong enough to destroy her ovaries' function, she would never begin to menstruate. Such a young woman could take hormones to bring on the changes of puberty, such as breast development and pubic hair, but would be unlikely to conceive or bear a child. Even after puberty, younger age is an advantage in preserving fertility. Research on women treated for Hodgkin's disease suggests that women who are under age 20 at the time of radiation therapy are more likely to keep on menstruating (and, thus, to be fertile) than are older women.

Chemotherapy and Women's Fertility

Alkylating chemotherapy drugs (including cyclophosphamide [Cytoxan], chlorambucil, busulfan, procarbazine, nitrosoureas, nitrogen mustard, and l-phenylalanine mustard) are the ones most likely to damage women's ovaries. Either adjuvant chemotherapy for breast cancer or the combination of drugs used to treat Hodgkin's disease commonly include one or more alkylating drugs. On the other hand, good fertility is often seen in young women after platinum-based chemotherapy used to treat early-stage ovarian tumors.

The older a woman is at the time of her chemotherapy, the less likely she is to remain fertile. When women have alkylating drugs as part of their chemotherapy, many who are under age 35 keep or recover normal menstrual cycles. With higher chemotherapy doses, however, even a very young woman's ovaries may be damaged. Women who are over 35 may go into menopause even with just a medium dose of chemotherapy.

When alkylating drugs are given before the age of puberty, most girls menstruate normally and are fertile later on. Even in childhood, however, the ovaries sustain some damage from chemotherapy. The number of follicles decreases, and scarring occurs in the outer areas of the ovary. A decrease in blood supply to the ovary can also occur.

An additional risk is that young women who continue to menstruate after chemotherapy, or who recover menstrual cycles after a few months, may still become prematurely menopausal, typically when they are only in their twenties. This pattern has been observed in women treated for Hodgkin's disease. The risk of premature menopause in young women who stay fertile after chemotherapy for breast cancer or childhood malignancies is not yet known. Once menopause begins, even powerful fertility drugs rarely can stimulate a woman to ovulate, and her chance of conceiving is very poor. Currently, women who have had chemotherapy as children, teenagers, or young adults are advised to get pregnant as early as is feasible in their lives. They may not have the option of waiting until their late twenties or early thirties to have a child.

Preventing Infertility during Cancer Treatment

Researchers hoped that women's ovaries could be protected from radiation or chemotherapy by using hormones to shut down ovulation. Most trials have not been successful. Neither oral contraceptive pills nor other medications called luteinizing hormone releasing hormone (LHRH) ana-logues (such as Lupron or Goserelin) have been able to help preserve women's fertility.

Recently, an Israeli group reported much better success in protecting the ovaries by injecting women with a long-acting drug that produces a temporary menopause, starting before chemotherapy for Hodgkin's disease and continuing for up to six months. Some of the women also received radiation to their shoulders and upper abdomens (mantle field). In the group who had the drug, more than 90 percent resumed menstruating—a much larger percentage than in a group that had finished treatment just before the project began (fewer than 50 percent). These results offer real promise but need to be repeated in other centers.

Embryo, Egg, and Ovary Banking

A young woman who is married when her cancer is diagnosed may have the option of banking embryos before treatment through IVF. She would have to delay her treatment for a month or two while she took powerful hormones to stimulate her ovaries to ripen multiple eggs. Those eggs could then be retrieved in a minor surgical procedure called vaginal aspiration and fertilized with her husband's sperm. Any embryos that resulted could be frozen for future use. A single woman has the option of using semen banked from an anonymous donor to fertilize her eggs.

Embryo banking is not widely used, however. IVF is expensive, and there is a good chance that replacing the embryos will not produce a successful pregnancy. Delaying cancer treatment for a month or two may be risky in itself, depending on the type of malignancy. Results have also been disap-pointing because cancer itself sometimes interferes with a woman's response to the stimulating drugs.

A few women have an egg retrieval just before ovulation without going through hormone stimulation (natural-cycle IVF). Unfortunately, this usually means that only one ripe egg is available. The chances are small that it will be fertilized successfully, that the embryo will be frozen and thawed successfully, and that the embryo will then implant successfully in the woman's uterus during attempted conception.

A hope for the future is that egg banking will become feasible. A woman would be able to have a piece of her ovary removed before cancer treat-ment. A good number of unripe eggs could be frozen and banked. Later, when she was ready to become pregnant (or perhaps had another woman willing to serve as a gestational carrier—see Chapter 22), her eggs could be thawed, ripened in the laboratory, then fertilized with her partner's sperm, and placed in her uterus.

A few pregnancies have recently been achieved using *mature* eggs that were frozen, thawed, and then fertilized with semen in vitro. Egg freezing is still not perfected, however. A further step will be to ripen *immature* eggs successfully before *or* after freezing. Research is ongoing, and egg banking is likely not very many years away.

Recently, the Genetics and IVF Institute in Fairfax, Virginia, began to advertise ovary freezing before cancer treatment. They offer an experimental program that involves surgically removing one ovary (or occasionally both) if cancer treatment such as a bone marrow transplantation is likely to destroy ovarian function completely. The *cortex* (the outer part of the ovary that contains the eggs) is cut into thin strips and frozen. In animal experiments using mice and sheep, these strips of ovary have been thawed and replaced surgically near the fallopian tubes. New blood vessels grow to supply the ovarian tissue. Pregnancies have occurred in sheep, and the tissue has produced hormones. This treatment could theoretically offer both a chance at fertility and at reversing premature menopause. The fertility experts would work with a woman's oncologist to determine when it would be safe to restore the ovarian strips. If techniques improve for thawing and maturing individual eggs in the laboratory, oocytes in the stored tissue could also be used for that purpose.

This advertisement sparked a good deal of controversy, and the American Society for Reproductive Medicine sent out a bulletin to its members reminding them that ovary freezing is totally unproven in humans and should only be offered as part of a research project. Unfortunately, women who want to participate in this research may have to pay several thousand dollars in medical costs, unless the researchers have funding to cover the surgery and storage fees. It is important to realize that freezing a piece of ovarian tissue may well be a waste of effort and money with the limited knowledge we have today.

Treatments to Enhance Ovulation after Cancer

Infertility treatment after cancer is often limited because techniques to stimulate better egg production do not work well in a damaged ovary. If chemotherapy or pelvic radiation therapy shut down the ovaries completely, even powerful drugs used to stimulate ovulation are ineffective. Women who are left with irregular menstrual cycles after cancer treatment may have some ovarian reserve left. They may be candidates for drugs such as clomiphene (Clomid, Serophene), human menopausal gonadotropin (Pergonal or Humegon), or FSH (Metrodin). If attempts at pregnancy through natural intercourse are not a success, these drugs are often combined with intrauterine insemination, or IVF is offered (see Chapter 18).

A recent study suggested that women who take clomiphene for more than twelve cycles may increase their lifetime risk of ovarian cancer. Scientists also suspect a link between ovarian cancer and the stronger drugs used in infertility treatment. The debate continues, however, with another recent paper suggesting that women at risk for ovarian cancer are more likely to have ovulation problems. Because these women would have a higher chance of ending up on fertility drugs, their increased cancer risk, rather than the drugs themselves, may explain the greater rates of ovarian cancer in groups of infertile women. Most women with a history of cancer do not have any special risk for ovarian cancer, which strikes one in seventy women on the average. A few women may inherit a gene that greatly increases their risk of ovarian cancer. A woman with a strong family history of breast or ovarian cancer should think carefully about taking fertility drugs, although their impact on women who carry a gene for ovarian cancer risk is unknown.

Although men's fertility problems end with conception, women's concerns continue throughout a pregnancy. The next chapter discusses what is known about pregnancy after cancer treatment.

20

Pregnancy and Cancer: What Are the Risks?

Women who have survived cancer treatment and are able to conceive a pregnancy often worry about the health risks for themselves.

Risks of Triggering a Return of Cancer

In past years, pregnancy after cancer was often discouraged out of fear that it could stimulate cancer to reoccur. For most types of cancer, including melanoma and leukemia, current research suggests that pregnancy does not increase the chance of recurrence. Women with a history of breast cancer have a special concern, however, because of the fear that the high estrogen levels during pregnancy could stimulate any remaining cancer cells or start a new cancer growing. (For a detailed discussion of pregnancy and breast cancer, see Chapter 23.)

Women are often advised to wait two years after cancer treatment before trying to get pregnant. The main rationale for a waiting period is that most recurrences of cancer happen within two years. If a woman gets through this time without a return of cancer, her long-term survival is more secure.

General Health Risks of Pregnancy after Cancer

Certain types of radiation therapy or chemotherapy can damage a woman's heart or lungs, making the physical stress of pregnancy potentially dangerous. If a woman has had chemotherapy or radiation, her heart and lung capacity should be evaluated before she makes a decision to conceive. If damage is slight, a pregnancy may be possible, but with careful monitoring.

Radiation can also damage a woman's uterus, making the walls tougher and less able to stretch during pregnancy. Women who had radiation therapy to the abdomen (e.g., for Wilm's tumor of the kidney in childhood or for Hodgkin's disease) may be able to get pregnant, but they have a higher rate of miscarriage or of giving birth to low-birth-weight babies. (Low birth weight is associated with a greater risk of infant death or problems in development during childhood.) Women who have had radiation therapy and want to become pregnant should find an obstetrician who specializes in high-risk deliveries.

When a Woman Is Already Pregnant at Cancer Diagnosis

If a woman is diagnosed with any type of cancer during a pregnancy, the need to protect her health may outweigh the risks to her unborn child. If the pregnancy is in the first trimester and she has an aggressive cancer, she may be told that having an abortion and starting chemotherapy is her best chance for survival. If the pregnancy is in the second or, especially, the third trimester, chemotherapy may be given, although there is still a risk that it could cause birth defects. More commonly, the baby may be born prematurely or does not gain a normal amount of weight in the last stages of the pregnancy. Chemotherapy can also affect development of the fetal brain.

Radiation therapy during pregnancy is even more dangerous than chemotherapy to the fetus. If a localized breast cancer is found during pregnancy, a mastectomy is usually performed because this surgery and anesthesia rarely cause miscarriage or harm the fetus. Partial mastectomy would not be recommended unless it is late in the pregnancy because this surgery should be followed as soon as possible with radiation therapy.

> Louise had wanted to be a flight attendant since she was a child. An army brat whose family moved around the country, she had a yen for travel. She did fulfill her dream and worked for a major airline for ten years after college. In the course of that time, she met a businessman and married. At age 34, she was ready to start her family. When she was only three months pregnant, Louise felt a lump in her left breast. Her gynecologist was concerned and scheduled her to have a needle biopsy. Louise could not believe it when cancer was diagnosed. Nobody in her family had ever had breast cancer, and it was the last

thing she expected. Louise's husband's first concern was for her health, and he urged her to consider terminating the pregnancy. Her medical team reassured the couple, however, that Louise could safely have a mastectomy and continue her pregnancy, although breast reconstruction would have to wait until after delivery.

Although it was hard for Louise to feel lucky, she was tremendously relieved when all of the lymph nodes removed were negative for cancer. The rest of her pregnancy was a time of mixed emotions. She grieved for the loss of her breast but looked forward to her baby. She yearned to be a mother but worried about whether she would live to see her child grow up. At the end of the nine months, Louise delivered a healthy, six-pound son. She had always wanted to breast-feed her baby, and her oncologist encouraged it because breast-feeding might possibly decrease her risk of ever developing a tumor in her remaining breast. Louise successfully breast-fed for six months, although she had to do some supplementing with formula. When her son was 18 months old, Louise had a flap breast reconstruction. Because of her cancer history, she did not want another pregnancy and so felt comfortable using some abdominal tissue to form her new breast. Her surgeon did mention, though, that some women had carried pregnancies successfully after this type of surgery. Having the reconstruction helped Louise feel more like a normal woman and reduced the number of times in a day that she thought about her breast cancer.

What about the children born to cancer survivors? The next chapter reviews what we know about their health and about their own cancer risk.

21

Postcancer Kids: Are They Healthy?

Cancer survivors often worry about the health of their postcancer children. They fear that a child conceived after radiation therapy or chemotherapy will be born with a deformity or disability. They also wonder if their children are at increased risk of cancer in the future.

As we saw in the last chapter, giving radiation therapy or chemotherapy to the mother can damage the developing fetus during pregnancy, especially in the first trimester. In severe cases, the pregnancy often miscarries. When the pregnancy continues, however, most children appear healthy at birth. Dr. John Mulvihill of the University of Pittsburgh Cancer Center is keeping a registry of children exposed during pregnancy to cancer treatment (see Resources under Information Networks)—the information gathered about their health can help doctors counsel couples in the future.

Risk of Birth Defects in Children of Cancer Survivors

There is little evidence that cancer treatments cause birth defects in children conceived *after* the treatment. A large study of children born to survivors of childhood cancer found a rate of birth defects of about 4 percent, no different from that expected in the general population. The percentage of sons versus daughters born to this group was also normal.

Today, men or women who have survived cancer are told to go ahead and try for a pregnancy. *Amniocentesis* (sampling fetal cells in the amniotic fluid through a needle inserted through the mother's abdomen at around fourteen to sixteen weeks of pregnancy), chorionic villi sampling (CVS—a test similar to amniocentesis, but done earlier in pregnancy), or other methods of diagnosing abnormalities in a fetus are only recommended if risk factors other than cancer treatment are present (e.g., if the mother is over age 35, increasing her risk of a child with Down's syndrome). The true relationship of cancer treatment to birth defects is still hazy, however, because it would take detailed records of thousands of births to rule out a small increase in a particular type of birth defect. Women who took the chemotherapy drug Dactinomycin should be aware that it is suspected to cause abnormal fetal heart development. These women may want to have a fetal ultrasound or echocardiograph during pregnancy to make sure the fetal heart is normal.

Cancer Risk in the Children of Cancer Survivors

A concern more pressing than birth defects is the possibility that the child of a cancer survivor could be at risk for developing a related type of cancer someday. All cancers result from damaged genes, or *mutations*—damage that is caused by the environment or damage that is inherited.

What Is a Gene?

A gene is a string of chemical code made up of four kinds of deoxyribonucleic acid (DNA) molecules. This code acts as a blueprint to produce a chemical called a protein. Proteins control a cell's function and growth. In each and every cell in the body, a complete copy of human genes normally exists. The genes inside any one of your cells contain all the information needed to build a unique human being—you. Genes are located on small rodlike bodies called *chromosomes*. You receive two copies of each of your genes (except some of the genes on the X and Y chromosomes that determine your gender).

Genes not only guide the growth and development of a fetus; they also control the way a person's cells work all of his or her life. Each cell has its own special job—a heart cell makes chemicals that are very different from those produced by a brain cell. Thus, as a person grows, only some genes need to be active in each kind of special body cell. The rest of the genes are inactive, or turned off.

Environmental Damage

Most types of cancer are not inherited. They are caused by exposure to the environment during a person's lifetime. Sunlight, toxic chemicals, radiation, and some of the body's own chemical products are all able to cause gene damage. But unless a child was exposed to the same environmental damage before birth or shared with a parent a common environment that increased cancer risks (i.e., living in a house with high radon levels or being exposed to secondary cigarette smoke), the child would not be at increased risk for cancer, despite the parent's health history.

Inherited Damage

Some gene damage is inherited at conception. The bad copies of the genes can come from either parent or from both parents. Most genes known to increase cancer risk are *autosomal dominant* (i.e., they are not on the X or Y chromosome and one damaged copy of a gene is enough to cause a health problem).

Scientists believe that about 10 percent of breast and ovarian cancers, prostate cancers, and colorectal cancers involve an inherited defective gene. Several types of cancer may cluster in a family at risk. Breast and ovarian cancer are particularly likely to occur in the same family. Rarer types of cancer with an inherited factor include some Wilm's tumors (a childhood cancer of the kidney), retinoblastoma (a childhood cancer of the eye), malignant melanoma, and the Li-Fraumeni syndrome, in which breast cancer, leukemia, brain tumors, and sarcomas can occur within one family. Researchers suspect that some cases of Hodgkin's disease also have a genetic linkage in families.

When cancer is related to an inherited gene, it tends to occur at an earlier age than usual. Inherited breast cancer is often diagnosed before age 50, and inherited prostate cancer before age 55. In an organ that comes in pairs, for example two breasts or two eyes, inherited cancer is more likely to occur on both sides (bilateral).

Your Risk for Inherited Cancer

Your personal risk of getting cancer depends on your inherited genes and on the environmental risks you encounter during your life. Even people who have an inherited gene that puts them at high risk for cancer may escape the disease if they lead an unusually healthful life.

If you are wondering whether your family has a high risk for some type of cancer, the more information you have about your relatives and their health histories, the better. If you have relatives with cancer, it is important to know how old they were when the cancer was diagnosed. Exactly what type of cancer did they have? If cancer occurred in a twinned organ (like the eye or breast), did both organs have the cancer (bilateral tumor)? It may help to draw a family tree as in Figure 21.1. Use circles for women and squares for men. Try to include all your relatives, beginning at least with your grandparents, and including aunts, uncles, first cousins, and your own children. Color in the shapes that represent relatives with cancer. Put a slash through the names of relatives who have died. For relatives with cancer, write below their entry their age at the time of diagnosis and the type of cancer.

Do you see patterns in your family? High-risk families, like the one in Figure 21.1, will often have three or more cases of breast and/or ovarian cancer or of colorectal cancer. If you have a small family, however, even

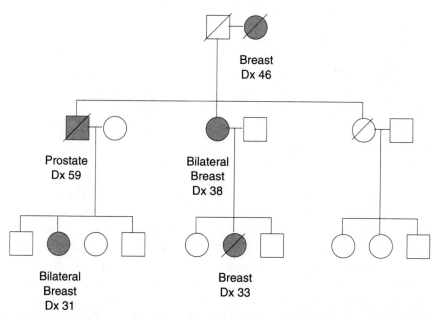

Figure 21.1 Family tree showing inherited cancer

one case of cancer of a type that is often related to inheritance and has been diagnosed at an unusually young age may be important.

If you think a gene for cancer risk runs in your family, you may want to contact a cancer registry that keeps confidential records and offers information and counseling for high-risk families. A registry will typically offer you suggestions for cancer surveillance—types and frequencies of special diagnostic tests to find cancer early. You may get advice on changing your lifestyle to minimize environmental cancer risks. You should also be informed about current programs of *chemoprevention* (medications that are under study to see if they reduce cancer risk). Registries often provide information about preventive surgeries (e.g., removing breasts, ovaries, or colon) to stop cancer from developing. You will want to become an educated health care consumer, keeping up with advances in our knowledge about genes and cancer.

Genetic Testing for Cancer Risk

For some types of inherited cancer, genetic testing is available to identify family members who have inherited the gene that puts them at risk. Before you make a decision about having genetic testing, you should receive counseling about the value of the information to be learned for your personal situation. Unfortunately, even people who know they carry a gene for cancer risk are left with difficult medical choices. Typically their most important safeguard is to have frequent screening tests to detect any developing cancer at an early stage. We do not know whether preventive surgeries, such as removing the breasts or ovaries, will actually prolong people's lives.

Currently there are few laws regulating genetic testing. Insurance companies may not cover genetic testing costs, and some have used inherited cancer risk as a basis to deny insurance coverage or to claim that a cancer that developed was a "preexisting condition" not covered by insurance. Employers could use this type of information to discriminate in the workplace, although the Americans with Disabilities Act guidelines forbid using a genetic risk for illness in making hiring or firing decisions. An employer could still limit or deny insurance for the illness if the company has its own self-insured plan, however. Thus, you take some risks in having genetic testing. If you try to conceal information from your insurance carrier, you could have your policy canceled or even be accused of fraud if the deception came to light.

If you do decide to have genetic testing, you should also receive personal feedback and psychological counseling when your test results become available and at scheduled follow-up times to ensure that you have a clear understanding of your situation and feel comfortable emotionally. Your test results and emotional reactions are confidential, and medical personnel should not discuss them with your family members without your permission. Some family members may choose to have joint counseling sessions, however. Genetic counseling can help a couple to decide whether to conceive a child who may be at risk for cancer or to learn how to best protect the children they already have.

In most cases, genetic testing is not performed on children under age 18 because the child cannot give informed consent. An exception is the inherited disease Familial Adenomatous Polyposis (FAP) in which hundreds of colon polyps develop during late childhood and early teenage years. Children need to be screened for polyps beginning at age 10, and they usually have surgery to remove the entire colon by the time they are young adults. In the case of FAP, a genetic test showing that a child has not inherited the disease lets a family avoid uncomfortable and expensive medical examinations.

Genetic testing for cancer risk may be available in the near future for the unborn fetus. Cells from the fetus could be gathered for genetic testing early in pregnancy through procedures like amniocentesis or CVS. Obviously this raises many ethical issues. Is it right to abort a fetus carrying a gene for cancer risk if there is a chance that this individual will never develop the disease? Perhaps by the time this potential child grows up, cancer will be far more easily detected and treated. On the other hand, what is the impact on a child of growing up in dread of cancer at an early age? Can't a woman who has seen half her family members mowed down prematurely by cancer exercise the right to bear a child who is not at risk?

Couples who would not consider abortion sometimes are more comfortable with preimplantation genetic diagnosis (testing embryos produced through IVF for a defective gene). In this amazing procedure, one cell is taken from each developing embryo and tested for a gene mutation. Only the embryos that do not carry the defective gene are transferred into the mother's uterus. This technique has already been successfully used for couples at risk to have a child with cystic fibrosis or Tay-Sachs disease, but it is still very difficult technically and experimental. Neither prenatal nor preimplantation genetic tests are yet available for cancer risk genes.

Genetic counseling for cancer risk is a very new area of medicine, and not every city will have a hospital offering these services. You can get more information about genetic testing by calling the National Society of Genetic Counselors (see Resources under Information Networks).

Melissa lived with the fear of cancer since her early childhood. Her mother died at age 36 of ovarian cancer. Melissa was only 5 at the time. Her mother's sister, Eileen, took a very active role in caring for Melissa and her older sister, Lynn. Eileen was diagnosed with cancer first in one breast and then in the second before she reached 35. She died when Melissa was 12. Then, worst of all, Lynn got breast cancer at age 27. Although her tumor was found at an early stage, and she survived her surgery and chemotherapy, Lynn chose to have her second breast and her ovaries removed in the hopes that she could avoid a second malignancy. Lynn was closer to Melissa than anyone else on earth. The two sisters had looked out for each other through their childhood losses. Lynn had one daughter, who was also the apple of Melissa's eye.

Melissa herself married in her midtwenties but told her husband ahead of time that she probably did not want children. She doubted she would live to see 40 and did not want to put a child through the trauma of having a parent with cancer. Melissa was 32, still with no sign of cancer, when she heard that a large cancer center in her city had started a program for women at high risk of breast cancer. The nurse at the clinic was excited to hear about Melissa's family history and asked if Lynn and their one surviving maternal aunt would be willing to give blood samples for a research project on inherited breast and ovarian cancer.

Several months later, the nurse called Melissa. "You may have heard that the gene BRCA1 for inherited breast and ovarian cancer has been identified," she began. Melissa had indeed been following the news reports. "We have some information about BRCA1 in your family and wondered if you were interested in the results, with some genetic counseling, of course."

Melissa was afraid. Although she had always believed she carried the bad gene, hearing it out loud might be more than she could bear. She talked about her feelings with her husband and Lynn. They urged her to find out her results. Melissa thought for a few more days and decided to have the counseling and test results. Her husband and Lynn went with her to the session where she would be informed whether she carried the mutated gene. Melissa was astonished and burst into tears when she was told she did not carry the gene. Her risk of breast cancer was similar to other women without a family history—about one in eight chances in her lifetime. Because she did not have the mutated gene, she could not pass it down to any children she might have.

Although Melissa did indeed eventually decide to have a child, it took her about six months to feel ready. She was surprised by the degree of guilt she felt. She would survive, while Lynn, and perhaps Lynn's daughter continued to be at risk. It did not seem fair to Melissa, and sometimes she wished she could change places with the other women she loved. Melissa had some psychotherapy to deal with her feelings about the cancer in her family and to adjust to the fact that she was not doomed. When Melissa's own daughter was born, she named her Ellen, after her aunt yet with a small difference—a few undamaged fragments of DNA.

One way to avoid transmitting a gene for cancer risk is to have a child using a donated egg or sperm. The next chapter discusses a variety of types of third-party reproduction that are options for cancer survivors.

22

Having Whose Baby?
Third-Party Reproduction

There are a number of situations in which a cancer survivor's options for having a child could involve a person other than the survivor and partner. This chapter discusses sperm and egg donation, surrogacy, and adoption after cancer.

Using Sperm from a Donor

Using donated sperm to conceive is an option if a man no longer produces healthy sperm cells or if a couple does not feel ready for the expense and effort of in vitro fertilization with intracytoplasmic sperm injection (IVF-ICSI). Donated sperm can also be used to avoid transmitting a genetic risk from the husband.

Donor insemination has been used as an infertility treatment since the 1920s. Currently it is estimated that about 30,000 babies a year are born in the United States through donor insemination. Traditionally, families that used donated sperm have been advised not to tell children about their biological parentage, but to let them believe that they were the genetic offspring of both mother and father. The wish for privacy made it difficult for researchers to study the impact of donor insemination on families, but it is known that the parents of children born from donor insemination have divorce rates similar to other couples and that the children appear to be healthy and to do well in school. A recent study in England compared families who used a sperm donor with similar groups who had children through IVF, through adoption, or without any infertility problems. The children conceived with donor sperm were just as well adjusted and close to their parents as their peers. In fact, no matter what route it took to have a child, parents who had dealt with infertility felt more positively about their relationships to their children than did those couples who had offspring without a struggle. More couples today consider telling a child about using donor insemination.

Sperm donors in the United States are typically college or graduate students whose motivation is primarily financial. They may earn up to $3,000 over a period of months for donating their sperm through mastur-bation in the laboratory. If you are considering donor insemination, check the source of the semen to make sure it comes from a sperm bank that is certified by the American Association of Tissue Banks. Sperm donors are carefully screened medically. Besides gathering a family health history, some sperm banks test for a few genetic diseases. Screening for sexually trans-mitted diseases is especially rigorous. The guidelines of the American Society for Reproductive Medicine only allow frozen and thawed semen to be used for donor insemination. The donor is tested for HIV and other sexually transmitted diseases (STDs) when he enters the program. His semen will not be used until a repeat HIV blood test is obtained, six months after his last donation.

Almost all donors in the United States give semen with the assurance that their identities are sealed. Like adoption, however, it is possible that laws in the future will unseal these records. It is rare in the United States to use a donor who is known to the couple. Occasionally a family mem-ber, such as a brother or father, may donate semen. A very few sperm banks also offer donors who are willing to have their identities known to a child in the future. Most typically, the information available about a donor includes his ethnicity, coloring, height and weight, and education or pro-fession. A recent trend is to offer couples more information about a donor's personality or talents, but only a few sperm banks provide this extra pro-file.

Donor insemination is medically very simple. The woman who will carry the pregnancy is inseminated in the doctor's office. Most inseminations involve placing the semen into her vagina or directly into her uterus when she is at her most fertile time. Ovulation kits are typically used to time the insemination. If the woman has had some fertility problems herself, she may be given hormones to enhance her ovulation.

Donor insemination is regulated by law in most states. In a married couple, the husband assumes legal fatherhood when he signs the informed consent form to use donor insemination. The donor is not held legally responsible for any offspring who result.

Using Eggs from a Donor

The use of donated eggs, or oocytes, is a much more recent option that can give a woman with damaged or absent ovaries but a healthy uterus a chance to carry a pregnancy. A healthy young woman gives her eggs to the woman with a fertility problem. The donor's eggs are fertilized with sperm from the husband of the infertile woman. Fertilized embryos are then transferred into the infertile woman's uterus.

Although egg donation involves IVF, the woman who carries the pregnancy does not have to take powerful drugs to stimulate her ovulation. She does take estrogen and progesterone to prepare her uterus to receive the embryos and to maintain the early pregnancy if an embryo implants. We do not know whether it is as safe for a woman with a cancer history, particularly breast cancer, to carry a pregnancy from egg donation as it is to have to a natural pregnancy. Because the artificial hormone levels are designed to mimic those of natural pregnancy, the risks are probably similar.

Like semen donors, egg donors are carefully screened for genetic risk and STDs. An egg donor must go through a much more unpleasant and medically risky procedure than a semen donor. Like a woman who has IVF, the egg donor must take strong hormones to stimulate ripening of multiple eggs and then have a small surgery to retrieve her eggs—a needle, guided using an ultrasound image, passes through her upper vagina and into the ripe follicles.

It is not always easy to find egg donors. Many clinics ask a woman to bring a sister, relative, or friend as her donor. Others will find a woman who will donate her eggs in return for some financial payment for her time and trouble. Donors may get from $1,200 to $6,000 a cycle. Research shows that most anonymous donors are primarily motivated to help the infertile couple. Perhaps because they typically are paid much less than a semen donor for a much more difficult task, they tend to be more altruistic. Egg donors are often older than semen donors, in their midtwenties to early thirties. Many clinics require that the donor has had a child herself because she is potentially endangering her own future fertility. If a volunteer donor is used, some clinics want the donation to be anonymous, with no contact between the couple and the donor. Others allow the couple and donor to meet.

There are few state and no federal laws regulating egg donation. Most couples simply put the birth mother's name on the birth certificate.

With a known donor, there is always a small risk of a court case, with the donor claiming some parental rights. Anonymous donation gives more protection to the couple. The American Society for Reproductive Medicine advises that all participants in egg donation have psychological counseling to make sure they are comfortable with their choices and that the donor has not been coerced by money or family pressure.

In 1994 in the United States and Canada, 2,587 cycles of egg donation were performed with anonymous egg donors and 532 with known donors. The birth rate per egg retrieval was 47.8 percent for anonymous donation and 42.1 percent for known donation, over twice the success rates for IVF using a woman's own eggs. Success is so high because egg donors are typically young and healthy, without a history of fertility problems. In addition, the uterus of the woman who will carry the pregnancy is optimally prepared with hormones and has not been affected by the drugs taken to stimulate ovulation.

A cycle of egg donation can cost between $10,000 and $20,000, with no guarantee of pregnancy. Egg donation is typically not covered by insurance. Some policies cover part of the cost, for example, the medications, the ultrasound tests, or the embryo transfer. Most policies do not cover the expenses of the donor's care.

Because several embryos are transferred into the mother's uterus, there is at least one chance in three that a multiple pregnancy will result. Carrying more than one fetus increases the chance of miscarriage, giving birth prematurely, or having a low-birth-weight baby.

Ingrid had chemotherapy for Hodgkin's disease when she was 22. She recovered her menstrual periods for three years after her treatment ended, but she was never regular. When she was 26, her periods stopped altogether, and tests showed she was prematurely menopausal. Her gynecologist was able to prescribe estrogen and progesterone to prevent hot flashes and vaginal dryness, but blood tests showed that her ovaries were too damaged to respond to hormone treatment for infertility. Ingrid was lucky because her older sister, who already had two children, was planning to have a tubal ligation. The sister offered to go through a hormone stimulation cycle so that she could produce extra eggs that could be harvested during her operation. The eggs were fertilized in the laboratory with semen from Ingrid's husband. Six healthy embryos resulted, and three were transferred into Ingrid's uterus. Nine months later, she delivered healthy twins. Ingrid's family planned to be open about the egg donation and would explain it to the twins as soon as they were old enough to understand the story.

Surrogate Mothers and Gestational Carriers

Some women may still be able to produce eggs, but no longer have a healthy uterus or have other health risks that prevent carrying a pregnancy. These women and their husbands may want to unite their egg and sperm through IVF and have their embryos implanted in another woman's uterus. That woman would then become the *gestational carrier* of the pregnancy, although she would not be the genetic mother of the baby. In 1994, sixty-four infertility programs in the United States and Canada performed these procedures, resulting in seventy children born.

The most controversial type of third-party reproduction is having another woman, a *surrogate mother*, inseminated with sperm from the husband in the infertile couple (or sometimes with semen from a gay man who wants a child). Thus, she both contributes the egg and carries the pregnancy. Records are not kept nationally of the number of surrogate-mother births, but perhaps 1,000 such agreements occur yearly in the United States.

A few of these agreements occur within families, with a sister or mother carrying the pregnancy. More are legal contracts with a woman who is recruited by the couple or infertility program and agrees to carry the pregnancy for financial compensation. Some states have laws either validating or outlawing these contracts. Many states have no laws regulating the agreements. Most surrogates and gestational carriers are carefully screened by mental health professionals. They keep their side of the bargain and feel great satisfaction at having helped the infertile couple. The infertile couple also should participate in mental health counseling. Of course the few agreements that go awry are the ones that get publicized in the media. More information about surrogacy can be obtained through The Organization of Parents through Surrogacy (see Resources under Information Networks).

Dilemmas in Using Third-Party Reproduction

Society has not yet come to terms with third-party reproduction. Different groups have very different views on whether it is ethical or desirable. Choosing to use a donor or gestational mother is a very complex and personal decision. Some religious groups, such as the Roman Catholic Church, believe that third-party reproduction is morally wrong. Feminists worry that egg donors or surrogate mothers are being financially exploited as baby factories by wealthy women who can afford to hire their services. Mental health professionals worry about the unknown impact of these technologies on the children they create.

Couples who have faced the pain of infertility often have more open views than does the public at large. On the positive side, third-party reproduction allows a couple to experience pregnancy and ensure good prenatal health care. At least one partner ends up with his or her genetic child. For cancer survivors, who are often shut out of public agency adoption, the legal risks and financial burden of these brave new technologies may not be any worse than those attached to private or international adoption.

On the negative side, couples worry about whether the parent who has not contributed a gamete will bond equally with the baby. Some couples forgo gamete donation because it feels inherently unfair. Others see it as a kind of infidelity or betrayal of their marriage vows. A couple should not consider third-party reproduction until they have had a chance to discuss these concerns openly, preferably with the help of an expert mental health professional.

Perhaps the biggest dilemma is whether to tell the child about gamete donation. Mental health professionals worry that when gamete donation is kept secret, the child will sense that something is wrong or may find out the truth in some negative and shocking way. Arguments for openness with children are made with a great deal of passion within the mental health community. Studies of families that used donor sperm, however, have not shown any obvious ill effects of secrecy on the children. There is really no scientific basis to guide parents about openness, although some long-term studies of gamete donation families are now under way. Currently about a third of families who use donor semen in the United States plan to tell their child about it. A higher percentage of families who use donated eggs opt for openness, perhaps because women tend to be feel less private or stigmatized about their infertility. As the amount of genetic information increases in everyone's medical records, it may become much more difficult to hide gamete donation in the future.

If parents believe they may not wish to tell a child about the donor, the best policy is not to tell any other relatives or friends, either. Studies show that parents often later regret having told people about sperm donation because they know they have increased the risk that a child could find out about it from someone outside the immediate family. A couple can always decide to be open with a child; but once they tell others, they have closed off some of their options for privacy. One advantage of openness is that the couple can reassure their child that she or he has not inherited a gene that increases cancer risk. On the other hand, couples often worry that their extended families will disapprove of gamete donation and will not love and accept their child. In a family with very traditional ethnic or religious values, it may be best not to disclose the use of gamete donation.

If a friend or family member serves as donor, a concern is that he or she will want more influence in the child's life than is comfortable for the couple. Sometimes the donor may have different views than the couple on whether to tell the child about his or her genetic origins. These are thorny issues that should be discussed before deciding to use a known donor. Each party in the agreement, including the donor's spouse, should be interviewed and counseled separately by a mental health professional.

If a couple decides to be open, when and how should they tell a child? Each child is different, but telling a child about third-party reproduction should be done when he or she is old enough to understand how babies are conceived and born. Thus the story of his or her birth can be part of the child's education about sexuality and reproduction. Several helpful storybooks are available and can be ordered by mail from their authors or distributors (see Resources under Books).

Adoption after Cancer

The decision to adopt a child after surviving cancer is also a very personal one. Adopting a healthy infant has become increasingly difficult, not only in the Caucasian community, but also within many minority communities. Many public agencies are not willing to consider a couple if one partner has a history of cancer. Some are more open, however. If a number of years has passed since your cancer treatment and you have remained free of disease, you should ask your physician to write a medical letter about your excellent prognosis. Some cancer survivors also choose to conceal their health history from adoption agencies. Others may feel that their experience gives them special empathy and patience and may want to consider adopting a special needs child with a physical, intellectual, or emotional disability. Private adoptions are a choice for many couples as well, although they are more expensive and leave couples more legally vulnerable. International adoptions are another alternative. It is estimated that about 50,000 adoptions occur each year in the United States. (See Resources under Books and under Information Networks for several books and organizations, respectively, that provide helpful information about adoption.)

Men and women have a number of options for becoming parents after cancer treatment, including infertility therapy, third-party reproduction, and adoption. Choosing the strategy best for you may require individual soul-searching as well as sensitive and extensive communication with your partner. A mental health professional familiar with infertility can be a very valuable resource during this difficult process.

PART IV

SPECIAL STROKES
FOR SPECIAL FOLKS

23

Myths about Sex, Women's Health, and Breast Cancer

Because the original radical mastectomy was such a mutilating surgery, cancer specialists started worrying about the sex lives of women with breast cancer as long ago as the 1950s. A lot has changed since then. Today, for the one woman in eight in the United States who can expect to be diagnosed with breast cancer in her lifetime, mastectomy is no longer her only option, and rarely is surgery regarded as an emergency. Instead, she faces a bewildering array of choices about her cancer treatment, many with the potential to profoundly affect her sex life or (if she is among the 25 percent of women with breast cancer who are premenopausal) her fertility. You may think you know how breast cancer treatment affects sexuality, but as you'll see, many of the stereotypes about breast cancer and reproductive health are quite wrong.

Myth #1: Mastectomy Destroys Women's Sex Lives

Mastectomy has usually been presented in the media as ruining women's lives. The typical heroine is a cancer victim who considers suicide after her husband leaves her but resolves to go on alone, knowing that no man will ever want her again. Looking in the mirror will always be her worst nightmare. Baloney! Two recent large studies of women who had mastectomy for early stage breast cancer showed that, by a year after surgery, they were just as well adjusted emotionally and sexually as either healthy women or women who had surgery for benign problems. No unusual rates of divorce have been found after women get breast cancer.

Another comparison showed that women who choose to wear a breast prosthesis are just as satisfied with their body image as women who decide to have surgical breast reconstruction (although women who have reconstruction tend to be younger and more affluent as a group).

In fact, there is little evidence that losing a breast per se is the major source of women's distress about breast cancer. Only 10 percent to 20 percent of women with early stage breast cancer have major emotional problems. Women who have been depressed or anxious in the past are more vulnerable to the stress of cancer. Younger women are more upset, probably because cancer disrupts their lives more severely. Women who are unmarried and lack a network of supportive friends or family have more trouble coping. A major issue is the woman's prognosis. Women's lives and emotions are more severely affected when cancer cannot be controlled.

Myth #2: Women Who Have Lumpectomy or Breast Reconstruction Are Much Better Off than Women Who Have Mastectomy Alone

When a few pioneering physicians fought to get the medical community to accept lumpectomy as an alternative to mastectomy, they believed the new operation would make a vast difference in the quality of women's lives. Champions of breast reconstruction also had an uphill battle to convince their colleagues that women who wanted a new breast were not narcissistic whiners. Every woman diagnosed with breast cancer should have the opportunity to choose the least extensive breast surgery that is safe for her or to have reconstruction. Research on quality of life shows clearly, however, that the benefits of these options are very limited and specific.

More than twenty studies have now compared women who had mastectomy with women who had breast conservation (lumpectomy typically followed by radiation therapy to the breast). In several research settings, women even agreed to accept a treatment chosen on a random basis. Whether women choose their own treatment or leave the decision to their surgeons, the main benefit of breast conservation is that women feel more positive about their appearance. But they are not happier, more likely to stay married, more likely to be sexually active, or more sexually satisfied than women who have mastectomy.

Studies of women who have breast reconstruction have reached almost identical conclusions. Breast reconstruction makes women feel better about their bodies. They feel more whole, believe they look more attractive, and can wear a wider range of clothing styles. Reconstruction has few other, more general advantages, however. Surgeons used to worry that women who had breast reconstruction immediately, at the time of mastectomy, would be dissatisfied with the results because they had not lived without a breast. In fact, women are at least as happy with the results of immediate breast reconstruction as they are when the reconstruction is delayed for months or years.

What if a woman is told that her breast cancer can be treated equally effectively by breast conservation or mastectomy with breast reconstruction? Which kind of treatment is best sexually and emotionally? My colleagues and I at the Cleveland Clinic Foundation surveyed a large group of women who had undergone either breast conservation or reconstruction an average of four years previously. The reconstructions in the women we studied were done at the time of mastectomy, usually using a tissue expander (a silicone shell that is filled with saline solution over several months to stretch the available skin) or permanent silicone breast implants. The two groups of women, those with breast conservation and those who had reconstruction, did not differ on the average in their overall psychological adjustment to breast cancer, their body image, relationship happiness, sexual satisfaction, or frequency of sex. A majority of each group was happy with breast appearance in clothing and in the nude.

Women who had lumpectomy rather than breast reconstruction had one advantage, however. They were more likely to continue enjoying breast caressing as part of their lovemaking routine. This makes sense because women are more likely to have normal breast sensation after a lumpectomy. With total mastectomy, the nerve that carries sensation from the nipple is removed. After reconstruction, the skin usually feels numb at first, gradually gaining more feeling during the healing process. Nerves can also be damaged during lumpectomy, depending on the location of the tumor, but many women retain nipple sensitivity. Nipples can be rebuilt surgically, but sensation cannot be restored. Some women say, however, that they feel more pleasure with touch after a nipple reconstruction. Perhaps mental arousal improves when a woman feels that her breast is closer to normal.

Nancy had always loved breast caressing, from the time she first experienced it as a teenager. In fact, she was often able to reach an orgasm just from having a sexual fantasy and softly pinching her own nipples. Nancy's husband always joked that her sensitivity to breast caressing was very convenient because it only took a minute or two of foreplay to get her ready to enjoy intercourse.

When Nancy was diagnosed with breast cancer, her surgeon recommended a modified radical mastectomy rather than lumpectomy because her type of tumor put her at risk for developing new cancer cells in any remaining breast tissue. Nancy chose to have immediate reconstruction with a flap of muscle and skin from her belly. "I'll get a new breast and a tummy tuck at the same time!" she told her friends gaily; but inside, she was very worried about losing her sexual pleasure. The mastectomy was to be on her favorite side, where nipple caressing was the most erotic.

Nancy chose not to have surgery on her opposite breast, even though her surgeon offered to lift it to match her reconstruction at the same time that he finished her nipple reconstruction surgery. She did not want to risk damaging sensation in her remaining breast. She continued to enjoy caressing on the side that had not undergone surgery but found little pleasure from touch on her reconstructed breast. Despite his teasing about minimal foreplay, Nancy's husband was very supportive about spending extra time on stroking and kissing other sensitive areas of her body to help her become aroused. Over time, Nancy was almost as easily orgasmic as before, but she still felt that losing a breast was a greater change for her than it would be for many other women.

Myth #3: A Woman Has Not Adjusted Well to Breast Cancer Unless She Learns to Love Her Scars

Many self-help books or magazine articles urge women to get used to their scars after breast cancer. Some feminists even advocate against wearing a breast prosthesis. I certainly agree that a woman can be beautiful without breasts and that it helps to get used to the changes in your body. You may want to practice looking at the area of your surgery in the mirror and gently touching yourself there. Some women find that, after healing, it helps to massage the breast area with body lotion as a way to get more comfortable with touch. Start with a short period of time and low lighting, and gradually increase your comfort level.

Some women find it hard to relax and enjoy sex with a partner, however, if their scars are exposed or caressed. Rather than try to adjust to nudity and direct breast caressing, they feel best when they camouflage their surgical scars, for example, by wearing a breast prosthesis with a camisole or bra for sex. They may prefer their lovers to skip any breast caressing, even on a side not affected by cancer. Each woman should use the strategy that works for her. There is no right or wrong. When first resuming lovemaking, a gradual approach using candlelight and starting with nongenital, sensual caressing may help you overcome anxiety about breast loss.

Myth #4: Silicone Breast Implants Are Unsafe and Should Be Banned Forever

Silicone-gel-filled breast implants provided a convenient and effective way to reconstruct the breast after mastectomy. In 1992, however, the Food and Drug Administration (FDA) began investigating reports that women who had silicone gel breast implants might be at increased risk for developing autoimmune diseases (illnesses in which a person's immune system attacks some part of her own body).

The most common type of disease seen in women with breast implants has been *scleroderma*. Its symptoms are joint pain and fibrous scarring of areas of the skin. Occasionally it affects vital organ systems such as the lungs. Other connective tissue diseases more rarely seen in women with breast implants include systemic lupus erythematosus and rheumatoid arthritis. In fact, most women who report ill health after breast implant surgery have symptoms such as fatigue, stiffness, muscle aches, and joint pain, but they do not have a clearly documented immune disease.

Great controversy remains about whether implants really cause autoimmune disease. Despite some large awards by juries to women for implant-related health problems, three large, recent scientific studies have not found such a connection. The University of Texas M. D. Anderson Cancer Center recently followed 250 breast cancer patients who had breast reconstruction using implants and 353 who had reconstruction using only their own tissue. Only one woman in each group had developed an autoimmune disease. The Mayo Clinic compared 749 women who had implants for various reasons to women in the community without implants but who were matched on other factors such as age and social class. Women with implants had fewer cases of connective tissue disease or arthritis than did the matched sample.

In the largest and most long-term study to date, researchers from Harvard studied 87,501 nurses from 1976 until 1990, before the scare about silicone implants became public. Within this group of women, 1,183 had breast implants and 516 had connective tissue diseases, but there was no relationship between the two health issues.

Several groups recently pointed out that the symptom picture of women with silicone-related disorders overlaps almost completely with two other fashionable but controversial diagnoses—chronic fatigue syndrome and fibromyalgia. It is unclear whether any of these disorders has a unique physiological basis or whether the symptoms represent a subtype of depression.

Manufacturers of silicone gel breast implants are currently doing studies of their safety. Meanwhile, gel implants are only available to women who have had a mastectomy in a few research centers. Implants that consist of a silicone shell filled with a saline solution are being used instead. Saline is a sterile saltwater solution that would not harm the body if it leaked. Although it is possible that the silicone shell could be a source of problems, most researchers believe that any health problems linked to implants are far more likely to be related to leaking silicone gel.

Saline-filled implants have some disadvantages, however. They do not feel as much like natural breast tissue as a silicone gel implant would. The saline sometimes sloshes with movement, a problem more noticeable to the woman herself than to those around her, but still uncomfortable. A certain percentage of the implants spring a leak and deflate over time. Leaks can only be fixed by taking the old implant out surgically and putting in a replacement. There are also concerns that the saline solution may become contaminated with bacteria.

Whether breast implants are made with silicone gel or saline inside, two other common drawbacks exist. As tissue around the implant heals after surgery, some women develop a contracture of the capsule, forming a hard envelope of scarring around the implant. The reconstructed breast feels overly firm and can be quite tender.

The other hazard is that the implant could interfere with finding new cancer cells after breast reconstruction. If breast cancer returns in the local area, early diagnosis and treatment is important. There is little evidence that silicone implants themselves promote breast cancer, but they do interfere with accurate mammograms. In many cases the implant can be squeezed aside to allow a good view of most remaining breast tissue, but some expertise is needed on the radiologist's part. It is rare to miss a breast cancer recurrence because a woman had a breast implant for postmastectomy reconstruction. Young women who have implants to enlarge their breasts, however, may jeopardize their chances of an early diagnosis of breast cancer.

If a woman can find a surgeon to implant a gel-filled implant, her decision should take into account the value she puts on a natural look and feel to her reconstructed breast as well as her estimation of the chance that she could develop implant-related health problems. Some women may elect to have a breast reconstruction using only their own tissue. Reconstruction with flaps of muscle and skin from a woman's belly or buttocks can produce excellent results. These surgeries are complex and expensive, however, and require a longer recovery than other types of reconstruction.

Myth #5: Prophylactic Mastectomy Ensures That a Woman Will Never Get Breast Cancer

As we identify the 10 percent of breast cancers that are related to a mutated gene (see Chapter 21), more young women with a strong family history of breast cancer are considering having prophylactic mastectomy, removal of both breasts to prevent breast cancer from developing. Because women who carry a mutated breast cancer gene are at risk for multiple breast tumors, women who have breast cancer at an early age and have a suspicious family history of cancer also may also consider having a full mastectomy on the side with cancer and a prophylactic mastectomy on the other breast. Do these operations make a woman safe from breast cancer for the rest of her life?

In the past, prophylactic mastectomy was often performed subcutaneously, removing breast tissue while preserving the skin and nipple. This operation leaves behind areas where a tumor could get started. In today's prophylactic mastectomy, the surgeon can spare a thin layer of skin but usually removes the whole nipple and as much breast tissue as possible. Even so, the risk of breast cancer remains at least 1 percent and probably more. We do not yet have any way of predicting whether prophylactic mastectomy will save lives of women who inherit a mutated breast cancer gene. As long as some breast tissue is present, cancer could develop. Many of these women have an increased risk of ovarian cancer as well. Another dilemma is that many insurance providers will not cover prophylactic mastectomy (which usually includes an immediate breast reconstruction). A woman who fights for coverage also alerts her insurer to her increased genetic risk—perhaps making her less insurable in the future if she switches policies.

We also lack knowledge about the impact of prophylactic mastectomy on women's quality of life. Are women more relaxed and less preoccupied with cancer risk after surgery? Do they still get their recommended mammograms and breast exams for cancer detection? Are their sex lives affected negatively? In the next few years, we will undoubtedly learn more.

For now, any woman considering a prophylactic mastectomy should look carefully at other options, for example, faithful and frequent cancer surveillance or participating in research on breast cancer prevention, such as the tamoxifen trial. Women who have not had breast cancer but have a suspicious family history should consider genetic testing before deciding on surgery because only half of women in the family will inherit the faulty gene. If a woman does not have a gene mutation, prophylactic mastectomy is less likely to be recommended.

Myth #6: Once You Are Through with Chemotherapy, It Has No Impact on Your Sex Life

Just as the sexual trauma of breast surgery has been overemphasized, the impact of chemotherapy has largely been ignored. Most women under age 50 with breast cancer are offered chemotherapy. The short-term side effects are well known: nausea and fatigue on and off for the months of treatment, hair loss, and weight gain.

The long-term side effects of chemotherapy are less often discussed but are quite significant. Most women over age 35 and many younger ones become permanently menopausal and infertile after chemotherapy. Unless they defy medical wisdom by taking replacement estrogen, their extra years of menopause increase their chances of developing osteoporosis and heart disease with aging. Chemotherapy also slightly increases a woman's lifetime risk of second malignancies.

What about the sexual side effects of chemotherapy? Surprisingly little is known about the impact of chemotherapy on women's sexual function, though vaginal dryness and pain related to premature menopause are certainly common (see Chapter 13). In a survey of women at an average of four years after treatment for early stage breast cancer, women who had chemotherapy had significantly more sexual problems and dissatisfaction than women who only had breast surgery and radiation therapy, and they were more likely to lose desire for sex, to have vaginal dryness and pain, and to discontinue sex. Those in the chemotherapy group also were more emotionally distressed and felt less attractive. I think evidence is increasing that chemotherapy is the breast cancer treatment most destructive to women's sex lives.

When women have lymph nodes that are positive for breast cancer, chemotherapy clearly increases survival time. More controversy arises when chemotherapy drugs are offered to women whose lymph nodes are all negative for cancer. Weighing a decision whether to have chemotherapy if you are in a group at low risk for breast cancer recurrence is difficult and very personal. If you have a very small breast cancer at the time of diagnosis and all your lymph nodes are negative for cancer, your chance of long-term cancer-free survival without chemotherapy is quite high—about 89 percent if the tumor is smaller than 1 centimeter and 77 percent when the tumor is 1 to 2 centimeters in size.

Try to imagine how you will feel if you refuse chemotherapy and one day become one of the 10 percent to 20 percent of women whose cancer returns. Will you blame yourself and feel you made a mistake? What if you choose chemotherapy and lose your ability to have a genetic child or to enjoy sex fully? Will the extra margin of safety make it worthwhile to you? Ask your oncologist to explain in detail what is known about your tumor's aggressiveness. Having that extra information may help you feel more comfortable with your choice.

Myth #7: Tamoxifen Causes Menopause and Other Sexual Problems

The drug tamoxifen (Nolvadex) often used to treat breast cancer is called an *anti-estrogen.* Women think of tamoxifen as a drug that causes menopause and interferes with sexual satisfaction. In reality, the story is more complicated. Tamoxifen does block the action of estrogen in breast tumors, but it behaves like a weak form of estrogen elsewhere in the body.

Tamoxifen does not make women menopausal. When young women take tamoxifen, only about 20 percent stop menstruating and another 25 percent have irregular menstrual cycles. Tamoxifen actually increases blood levels of estrogen in premenopausal women. Women are fertile while taking tamoxifen, but they are advised not to become pregnant because of a concern that the hormone could cause birth defects.

After menopause, women who take tamoxifen receive as a bonus some of the benefits of estrogen replacement. Like estrogen, tamoxifen prevents bone loss and has a positive impact on cholesterol. It also may help the vagina stay stretchy and produce lubrication.

Tamoxifen is suspected to cause depression in a minority of women and is often blamed for loss of sexual desire. The one research project that compared tamoxifen to a placebo (sugar pill), however, found it had a slightly positive impact on sexual desire. The sexual side effects of tamoxifen in healthy women who take it to prevent breast cancer are not yet known but are being monitored. Because women who take tamoxifen have often had chemotherapy, I believe that the sexual problems from chemotherapy are often attributed to tamoxifen. Tamoxifen does increase hot flashes, but otherwise may do little harm to women's sex lives.

Myth #8: Women Should Never Take Estrogen after Breast Cancer

Women who have had breast cancer have traditionally been told never to take any form of estrogen again. Many breast tumors grow in response to estrogen, so the hormone could cause the cancer to reoccur or advance. With new knowledge that estrogen replacement after menopause extends women's lives (see Chapter 3), physicians are beginning to question whether the benefits outweigh the risks for some women after breast cancer.

Some women are already using replacement estrogen, especially those free of cancer for several years whose tumors were small and localized. Some breast tumors do not have *receptors* for estrogen (chemical keyholes that allow estrogen to enter a cell), suggesting that hormones are less likely to influence growth of the cancer cells.

Follow-up studies of women who have risked taking replacement estrogen after breast cancer have not suggested any increased cancer recurrence or deaths so far. Larger scientific studies of the safety of estrogen replacement are just getting under way. Until we know more, each woman should discuss her individual situation with her physicians to make the most informed choice possible.

Myth #9: Women Should Never Risk a Pregnancy after Breast Cancer

In recent years, medical thinking about pregnancy and breast cancer has changed radically, as Table 23.1 shows.

Recent research suggests that a first pregnancy is a time of increased cancer risk in very young women diagnosed with breast cancer. One study of women under 30 found that those diagnosed during or soon after a pregnancy had poorer long-term survival. It is difficult to translate these findings into advice for women on having a pregnancy *after* breast cancer, however. For breast cancer survivors with localized tumors, studies have been reassuring that having a pregnancy after treatment has no impact on cancer recurrence or survival.

Table 23.1
Attitudes about Pregnancy and Breast Cancer, Past vs. Present

Past Thinking	Present Thinking
If breast cancer is diagnosed during a pregnancy, the woman will probably have a gloomy future.	Breast cancer is often diagnosed at a more advanced stage during pregnancy because the breast is more difficult to examine. Stage for stage, however, breast cancer diagnosed during pregnancy is as treatable as breast cancer in nonpregnant women of similar age.
If breast cancer is diagnosed during pregnancy, an abortion should be performed for the mother's safety.	Abortion is only recommended if a very aggressive cancer is found early in the pregnancy, when carrying the pregnancy to term would delay chemotherapy and possibly decrease the mother's chance of long-term survival.
If a woman has had breast cancer, she should never get pregnant again because it will increase her risk of the cancer recurring or of having a second breast cancer.	There is no evidence that a new pregnancy increases the risk of cancer recurrence or death, at least in women who had small tumors and negative lymph nodes.
If chemotherapy has created a premature menopause, no treatment options exist for infertility.	Women who have had premature menopause are excellent candidates to carry a pregnancy using an egg donated by another woman.
Women should not worry about passing breast cancer to their children.	Women who have breast cancer at an early age may carry a gene that would increase cancer risk in their children. Genetic counseling can be helpful in planning future pregnancies.

Women who have finished their breast cancer treatment and then get pregnant are often able to breast-feed if they have one breast that was not treated, or they even may produce milk from a breast that was treated with lumpectomy and radiation therapy. Breast-feeding may protect against future breast cancer because it causes the cells of the breast to specialize, making them more resistant to malignant changes. Breast milk from a woman who has survived breast cancer should not be harmful to her infant. Of course, women should not breast-feed during active chemotherapy treatment because some of the chemicals can be present in breast milk.

Being an Informed Survivor

Women with breast cancer have transformed their own images in the past fifty years, sharing information and support with each other and educating the public about the need for better breast cancer treatments. As more women have regular mammograms, breast cancer is being diagnosed earlier, and the image of the woman with breast cancer is changing from neutered victim to vibrant survivor.

The National Alliance of Breast Cancer Organizations (NABCO) publishes an annual list of resources, including educational materials, support groups, and advocacy organizations (see Resources under Information Networks). To keep up-to-date about breast cancer and your health, consider joining NABCO or ordering a copy of their Breast Cancer Resource List.

24

It's Not Prostrate Cancer

Although many men confuse the words *prostate* (the small gland underneath the bladder) and *prostrate* (flat on your face), prostate cancer survivors no longer are willing to take their cancer lying down. Taking their cue from breast cancer survivors, men have organized their own prostate cancer advocacy groups (see Resources under Information Networks). The sexual problems caused by prostate cancer treatments are some of the most important quality-of-life issues for survivors.

Choosing a Treatment for Localized Cancer: Weighing Survival and Sex

If you have to decide whether you want to have a cancer treatment that can save your life, but will also cause sexual problems, I do not see much of a dilemma. Unless you believe in heavenly hanky panky, you have to be alive to have sex! Choosing among the treatments for localized prostate cancer is a little more complicated, however. It is not always clear which treatment is most likely to save your life, and statistics about sexual problems after different treatments are often presented in misleading ways.

The Prostate Cancer Explosion

The number of men being diagnosed with prostate cancer that is still localized to the gland has increased radically since the blood test for *prostate specific antigen* (PSA), a chemical that warns of prostate cancer, has become widely used as part of a yearly cancer screening. In 1994, the American Cancer Society estimated that 200,000 new cases would be diagnosed in the United States. In 1995, the estimate was 244,000, a stunning 22 percent leap in one year. The average American male now has one chance in six of a prostate cancer diagnosis in his lifetime. African-American men are at particular risk for prostate cancer, with rates 30 percent higher than in Caucasian men.

Is Your Prostate Cancer a Sleeper?

Although early detection is crucial in treating cancer, experts question whether screening for prostate cancer is all to the good. In men over age 50, as many as a third of prostate cancers are of a slow-growing type that may never cause symptoms or be life threatening. A very high percentage of men in their eighties who die without any symptoms of prostate cancer actually have malignant cells in their prostate if an autopsy is done. If only these less troublesome tumors could be identified, many men could be spared the costs of cancer treatment, both in terms of dollars and reduced quality of life, including sexual problems. One way to handle this issue is to direct men into a program of *watchful waiting*—repeated prostate examinations, but no treatment unless the cancer advances.

Unfortunately, cancer cells tend to mutate and change over time, often becoming more abnormal. Tumors that look relatively nonthreatening can eventually spread and become lethal. Urologists believe that almost every prostate cancer would grow enough to cause health problems if a man lived long enough. Watchful waiting is offered to many older men with small, low-grade tumors, especially men over age 70 or who have less than a ten-year expected life span.

Will Nerve-Sparing Save Your Sex Life?

Most urologic oncologists favor radical prostatectomy to treat prostate cancers that have not spread beyond the gland itself, especially if a man is under age 70. With nerve-sparing surgery (see Chapter 10), surgeons also feel they can do a better job than their radiotherapist colleagues at preserving erections. But how often do men really recover good erections after nerve-sparing?

I think the percentages quoted in medical journals have been misleading. For example, a group of researchers headed by Dr. Patrick Walsh at Johns Hopkins interviewed more than 500 men who had recovered for at least eighteen months after radical prostatectomy. Sixty-eight percent were classified as *potent*. But what does *potent* mean? Dr. Walsh defined it as the ability to have an erection that allows a man to penetrate a partner's vagina and have an orgasm with his penis inside. In my experience, most men who seek help at a sexual dysfunction clinic could meet this standard: They get partial erections that are not really stiff. With effort they can just manage to "stuff" their penis into a partner's vagina, if she has good lubrication and is relaxed. Then they can thrust (very carefully, sometimes gripping their penis at the base with their hand) until they reach a climax. But these men are usually not very satisfied with their erections and want some treatment. When Dr. Walsh and his colleagues asked men if their erections were truly firm and normal, a much smaller percentage than the 68 percent answered yes.

Because Dr. Walsh and his group are famous for doing the best job possible of sparing nerves, they attract men from all over the world who want to preserve their sex lives when they find out they have prostate cancer. These relatively young, healthy, highly motivated men who seek Dr. Walsh are going to be more likely to recover erections after surgery. Several studies including a *broader* sample of men after radical prostatectomy show that erection problems are more common after nerve-sparing surgery than previously believed. One such study at the Dana Farber Cancer Institute in Boston included men from several large hospitals treated either with radical prostatectomy or radiotherapy. Another follow-up study of ninety-three men at the University of Wisconsin Hospital revealed that only 9 percent had full erections and 38 percent partial erections at an average of two years after their operation. In a survey of 255 managed-care patients with prostate cancer, only 20 percent of the surgery group reported that erections were fair to very good, compared to 30 percent of men who had radiotherapy and 39 percent who had watchful waiting.

Has Radiation Gotten a Bad Rap?

Radiation therapy has lost some popularity as a treatment for localized prostate cancer in recent years because of concern that it does not kill all the cancer cells. Biopsies of the prostate after radiation therapy often show remaining cancer. In the first five or ten years after treatment, surgery and radiation appear equally effective, but physicians worry that after fifteen or twenty years, cancer will again grow and cause problems in men who had radiation therapy, whereas men who had surgery may remain free of cancer.

On the other hand, when a tumor has spread to both sides of the prostate (Stage B2 or C), radical prostatectomy often leaves some cancer cells behind, limiting its curative impact. For men with larger tumors, radiation therapy may make sense as a first-line treatment. According to conventional wisdom, about half of men develop new erection problems after pelvic radiation for prostate cancer. Although we could use some better research, recent studies suggest that the risk of erection problems is less—perhaps only 25 percent. Men who have radiation therapy instead of surgery for prostate cancer are often older and in poorer health: just the guys likely to already have erection problems! Many of the older studies did not ask men about their sex lives before treatment, instead assuming that most problems after radiation were caused by the cancer therapy.

One type of radiation therapy that has much lower rates of sexual side effects involves implanting radioactive seeds or rods in the prostate. A network of radioactive seeds is placed in the prostate either surgically or, more recently, through needles from the anal canal, without need for an incision. This treatment provides a very high dose of radiation to a very limited area. The tissue around the prostate, including the blood vessels, does not get as much exposure to radiation as in the older techniques. However, whether these treatments are as effective as external radiation in controlling prostate cancer is controversial. Men with very large prostate glands may not be good candidates for seed implantation, nor would men who have already had transurethral surgery on the prostate.

Wallace was 72 when a mild elevation in his PSA blood test led his internist to send him for an ultrasound study of the prostate. A biopsy confirmed that he had Stage A2 prostate cancer of a grade that was called moderately well differentiated (i.e., medium in its speed of growth). Wallace's doctors suggested not treating the cancer at all, given his age. Wallace did not like the idea of having untreated cancer cells in his body, however. His brother had died of prostate cancer two years before, and Wallace remembered vividly how bone pain and weakness had affected his brother's last year of life. If treating the cancer might spare him a similar fate, Wallace was ready to undergo some discomfort. Besides, Wallace's parents had both lived to be over age 90, and he was healthy and active for his age. He felt he had longer than ten years left to enjoy his life. Wallace considered his choices and decided to have radioactive seeds implanted in his prostate. Wallace was a widower, but he had been dating a woman steadily for the past two years.

Although Wallace had some pain for several weeks after his surgery and went through a period of very frequent urination, these side effects mostly subsided after a month or two. His sex life changed very little. Having the radiotherapy helped Wallace feel he could put his cancer behind him.

An experimental treatment for prostate cancer is cryosurgery: In a surgical procedure, the prostate is frozen at extremely low temperatures to kill cancer cells. Currently, cryosurgery is used after radiation therapy has failed and medical tests show that cancer is growing again in the local area. In the future, cryosurgery may become a first-line treatment for localized prostate cancer. Cryosurgery does have the potential to damage the nerves involved in erection. In early reports, only about a third of men continued to have good erections after the procedure. Some additional men may recover better erections with healing during the first year or so after cryosurgery.

Erection problems after treatment for localized prostate cancer can be corrected (see Chapter 11). When prostate cancer has spread beyond the gland, the choices between sexual pleasure and survival become more painful.

Sex and Hormone Therapy: Making the Best of It

As we saw in Chapter 8, any type of hormone treatment for prostate cancer is likely to decrease a man's desire for sex, make it more difficult for him to get aroused, and interfere with erections and orgasm. But because there is no effective chemotherapy to treat prostate cancer, hormone therapy is the best game in town. For men whose cancer has spread beyond the prostate and who must have hormone therapy, there are still some choices to preserve sexual quality of life.

Many men these days have prostate cancer that is diagnosed through screening and is not causing any symptoms. If some cancer has already entered the lymph nodes, however, local treatment is not going to cure it. Many urologists believe that these men should start some type of hormone therapy as soon as possible, in the hopes that they will ultimately live longer. We have as yet only suggestive data showing that early hormone therapy prolongs life. When the results of large, long-term studies become available, more medical guidance will be available.

Currently the choice of when to begin hormone therapy is a matter of personal preference. A recent study from Memorial Sloan Kettering Cancer Center, however, found that men who delayed hormone therapy until the cancer was causing problems had better *quality* of life, including less fatigue, fewer bothersome physical symptoms (such as hot flashes), and better sexual desire and erections. These men, who were ready to take a risk, were no more anxious about their cancer during the time of the study than the men who decided to begin on hormones. The two groups of men were not followed for long enough to know if their survival time was different.

Another variation is intermittent hormone therapy. A luteinizing hormone releasing hormone (LHRH) agonist is used to bring a man's PSA down to very low levels. Then he takes a break from treatment, allowing his sex life to return to normal within several weeks. His PSA is monitored, and he resumes hormone therapy when it begins to rise.

Drugs (flutamide, Casodex) that block androgen hormones from entering their usual target cells are often added to LHRH agonists to control testosterone action as completely as possible. The androgen-blocking drugs can also be used alone, with fewer sexual side effects than other forms of hormone therapy for prostate cancer. The comparative long-term effectiveness of androgen-blocking drugs as a solo treatment is not yet proven, however. In a recent experimental study, men were put on a combination of flutamide and Proscar (finasteride) (see next paragraph). Early results look promising, in that the drug combination controlled the cancer but left 80 percent of men with normal sexual function.

Finasteride is also being studied in a large trial to see if it can prevent prostate cancer in men at high risk for the disease, and it is being used in men who have benign overgrowth of the prostate with aging. It helps to shrink the prostate and relieve difficulty with urination. Finasteride prevents the hormone testosterone from being changed to *dihydrotestosterone*, a stronger hormone that promotes growth of prostate tissue. Dihydrotestosterone may also act in the brain to promote sexual desire, but only a small minority of men (fewer than 5 percent) who start taking finasteride complain of new problems with reduced sexual desire or erections.

For large prostate tumors that are not yet in the lymph nodes, another frequent choice offered to men is radiation therapy versus hormone therapy. Although having radiation offers a man more chance to preserve his sexual desire, he does risk other side effects, such as urinary incontinence or damage to his bowel function.

The Trauma of Orchiectomy

A parallel between prostate and breast cancer is that mutilating surgery is sometimes used as a cancer treatment in both sites. *Bilateral orchiectomy*, the surgery to remove both testicles, used to be a more common way of getting rid of testosterone, before the LHRH agonist drugs became available. Some men still prefer to have a one-time surgery, instead of having to have a hormone shot once every month or every three months. I recently heard that some managed care companies push men to have orchiectomy because it is less expensive than long-term LHRH agonist treatment.

The kind of surgery that is performed for prostate cancer just removes the rounded bottom, or *capsule*, of each testicle. Because the cord that holds the testicle is left in place, a man's scrotum does not look totally empty. Many men still feel comfortable in a public men's room or locker room, but others are very self-conscious. Men who are single and would be dating new partners also worry about the impact of missing testicles. Men expect themselves to be comfortable with nudity in front of strangers and often feel ashamed of their distress.

Until recently, men had the option of having silicone gel-filled testicular implants placed in the scrotum when they had orchiectomy. These implants looked and felt like a testicle. When the controversy about breast implants began, however, the American Urological Association advised urologists not to use gel-filled silicone implants until safety studies could be completed. Autoimmune diseases are more rare in men than in women, and no case has been reported of a man getting scleroderma or rheumatoid arthritis related to a testicular implant. Because of the fear of lawsuits, however, the companies that manufactured silicone testicular implants have discontinued their products. Some may consider marketing them again in the near future, however.

Jorge was a 58-year-old Mexican-American elementary school teacher, married for thirty-six years when his metastatic prostate cancer was diagnosed. He was given the choice of orchiectomy or weekly hormone shots. Because Jorge lived in a rural Texan community, he decided surgery would be more practical. His wife could have learned how to give him injections, but Jorge had never liked needles. Jorge's coworkers and friends knew he had been to the city for cancer treatment, but he was quite vague in answering their questions about how he was feeling. He felt intensely shamed at the loss of his testicles. Even the priest at his church did not know what kind of operation Jorge had undergone.

Jorge not only did not approach his wife sexually, but he slept on the far edge of the bed instead of holding her close as he normally had. He stopped riding horses and taking walks in the fields. On weekends he mostly stayed in his woodworking shop. At school, Jorge had been a baseball coach. He asked to be relieved of this duty, citing health reasons. His real concern was that he did not want to change clothes or take showers in the locker room. Jorge's doctors had not mentioned testicular prostheses to him originally. When Jorge went back for a six-month follow-up visit, his wife came with him. With the doctor in the room, she described the changes in her husband's behavior and her concern that Jorge was deeply depressed. Jorge began to cry silently. "What do you expect?" he said softly. "I'm just not a man anymore."

Jorge's doctor tried to help him feel better about his cancer treatment, emphasizing the tumor shrinkage since his surgery. He mentioned that many men Jorge's age still managed to have a sex life and asked if Jorge would be interested in a penile prosthesis to give him better erections. "I don't care so much about that," Jorge said, "but I do wish I could have my testicles back. Every time I wash myself or get undressed, I feel that emptiness." Jorge's doctor suggested that testicular prostheses might help Jorge feel more whole again, even though they could not restore his sexual function. Jorge was interested in the idea of surgery, but he was reluctant to seek an operation just to improve his appearance. His wife convinced him by asking whether he would support her in getting a breast reconstruction if she ever needed a mastectomy. Jorge could easily see the parallels and did have testicular prostheses implanted. Knowing that his scrotum did not look empty, Jorge returned to more of his normal life. He expressed affection more openly to his wife, but they did not try sexual touching.

25

Sex with a Part Missing

Sometimes curing cancer means losing a vagina or a penis or having an ostomy to rid the body of urine or feces. It may be hard at first to imagine having a satisfying sex life under these conditions. Over my years of clinical experience, I have learned that people are amazingly resilient. If they have the will to have sex, they will find a way. The will to have sex, however, depends on overcoming grief and dismay at physical scars and having a partner who is loving and mature enough to value you as a whole person, not just a collection of body parts.

Radical Hysterectomy: Sex without the Uterus and Cervix

A number of self-help books and magazine articles warn women that having a hysterectomy can permanently damage their sexual pleasure. They predict disaster even after a hysterectomy for benign causes, much less the larger surgery that is done for cervical or uterine cancer. Typically these publications state that women need to have a cervix and uterus to experience a fully satisfying orgasm. Although the authors are usually well meaning, their claims are not based on scientific fact. Of course, if a woman's ovaries are removed at the time of her hysterectomy, she may have sexual problems related to an abrupt menopause. If a woman is under age 40, at least one ovary is usually left in place, even when she has a hysterectomy for cancer. Most women with cancer of the cervix or uterus can also take estrogen replacement safely if their ovaries are removed.

In my own research, I interviewed twenty-six women who were going to have radical hysterectomy for cervical cancer. This operation removes not only the uterus and cervix, but also ligaments that hold the uterus in place and the upper third to half of the vaginal canal. I asked the women about their sex lives at six and twelve months after their surgery. As a group, the women reported no change in their ease of reaching orgasm, whether from caressing around the clitoris or from intercourse. Only one woman said she felt her orgasm was weaker after surgery. Despite some loss of vaginal depth, few women experienced discomfort with intercourse by the time healing had taken place.

Women are more likely to have sexual difficulties when a combination of hysterectomy and radiation therapy to the pelvis is used to treat their cancer. This is a common treatment for cancer of the uterine lining. Typically women have pain during intercourse because of vaginal dryness or loss of vaginal size. The loss of vaginal size occurs because of a combination of surgical removal of the upper vagina and the impact of radiation in scarring the vaginal walls. Taking estrogen replacement can often help with the dryness and is considered safe for most women who had localized cancer of the uterus. (See Chapter 14 for other suggestions for overcoming painful intercourse.)

Donna sometimes felt jinxed. She never knew her father's identity, and her mother was killed in a car accident when Donna was 12. She was raised by loving grandparents, but she lost them both before she was 20. Nevertheless, Donna put herself through college and became a special-education teacher. She loved working with children who shared her African-American, southern background, and she always planned to have at least three kids of her own. She did marry when she was 25 to a warm and loving fellow teacher, Ronald.

Ronald and Donna wanted to start their family and were upset when no pregnancy had occurred after a year of trying. They consulted Donna's gynecologist, who did not find anything clearly wrong but tried her on hormones. Still Donna did not conceive, but she did have some unusual bleeding between her menstrual cycles. Concerned, she called her gynecologist, who did some tests and found that Donna had, at the unusually young age of 27, a localized cancer of the uterus. The only safe treatment was to have a hysterectomy. Because the tumor was still small, radiation would not be necessary.

Donna was devastated. Her aunts and cousins warned that Ronald might leave her, both because she would be "half a woman" without her womb and because she would not be able to give him children. To Donna, losing her dream of a close and loving family would be worse than dying. Ronald did his best to reassure his wife that he would always love and stand by her, even if they never had a child. As soon as she recovered from her surgery, Ronald began to cuddle close and gradually helped Donna feel ready to try sex. At first she cried during intercourse, not because of pain, but because of the thought that she and Ronald would never make a baby together. After time, however, sex felt just as loving and pleasurable as it always had.

Two years after her hysterectomy, Donna and her husband adopted a new-born boy. After a few months, neither partner believed they could have loved their own biological child more than they adored their son. Lovemaking remained a way that Donna and Ronald expressed their closeness and gave each other pleasure. As they both said, they never took each other for granted.

Radical Vulvectomy: Sex without a Vulva

Cancer of the vulva becomes more common with age, but sometimes it can be seen in young women. Vulvar cancer has a variety of causes. Just as the human papilloma virus (HPV) may promote cancer of the cervix, it may transform the skin cells of the vulva into a malignancy. HPV-related vulvar cancer is more common in women whose immune systems are not working well; for example, women who have had organ transplants and take drugs to suppress the immune system or women who have the human immunodeficiency virus (HIV). These vulvar malignancies are often found in an early stage, as carcinoma in situ, before they have invaded into the deeper layers of the skin. Carcinoma in situ of the vulva can usually be treated by removing the tumor and area around it with surgery. Although some tissue is lost, the clitoris and vaginal entrance usually remain and have normal sensation.

When vulvar cancer is more invasive, a larger surgery is often necessary. In radical vulvectomy, the entire vulva must be removed, including the inner and outer labia and the clitoris. The vaginal entrance may become narrowed by scar tissue after radical vulvectomy, and reconstruction with skin grafts is occasionally needed to make the vagina large enough for intercourse. A few surgeons have also used grafts made up of skin and underlying muscle from a woman's own thighs or belly to sculpt a new vulva for her. This kind of reconstruction can cushion the sensitive tissue around the urinary and vaginal openings and can give a woman a more normal-looking vulva; but the reshaped tissue will not have the same sensitivity as the woman's original vulva.

Another part of radical vulvectomy is removal of the lymph nodes that drain fluid from the vulva. Although the node dissection can be important in controlling vulvar cancer, it often leaves a woman with severe edema, or swelling, in both legs. The swelling is physically uncomfortable and also can be unsightly. Leg edema does not prevent a woman from having sex, but it can affect how attractive she feels.

Losing the vulva is traumatic. Women worry that they will no longer appeal to their lovers. Women who enjoyed having oral stimulation may lose their own pleasure in this activity and also fear that their partner will no longer find giving oral sex erotic. However, women who were sexually active before their cancer diagnosis often resume sex even after radical vulvectomy. Several studies have found that women can reach orgasm, even if the whole clitoris is lost. Some women have always been easily orgasmic from vaginal stimulation and continue that pattern after vulvectomy. Women who depended more on clitoral caressing may need to switch focus to pleasurable feelings inside the vagina, from breast caressing, or from gentle stimulation of the remaining tissue in the genital area. One survey of women after vulvar surgery found that the deciding factor in a woman's ability to resume an active and satisfying sex life after surgery was the quality of her close relationship, not how much tissue was removed from her vulva.

Gail's melanoma of the vulva was discovered two months after she married at age 21. She had also just finished nursing school. Her first concern with such a rare type of cancer was survival. Everything happened so fast that there was little time before surgery to think about quality of life. The doctors did tell the young couple that Gail could consider a pregnancy in the future, if her cancer did not return. She would probably have to have a cesarean section, however.

Once Gail was released from the hospital, she and her husband, Cal, were shocked by the extent of the surgery. They eventually were able to have intercourse, but Gail could not reach an orgasm.

Her leg swelling was so severe, even with special support stockings, that she could not tolerate a job that kept her on her feet all day. She had to switch to an administrative nursing job, even though she loved direct patient care.

It was only after three years of coping with these changes that Gail sought sexual counseling. She still missed the pleasure she used to feel in lovemaking. Cal came with her and was very supportive. Gail was so worried about disappointing him, however, that the therapist and couple decided to focus first of all on helping Gail to learn to get more pleasure from her own self-touch.

Gail practiced a couple of hours a week in privacy, reading erotic stories and gently caressing her remaining vulvar area. She used a water-based lubricant on her fingers to minimize irritation. She found two areas were more sensitive than she had realized: the remaining tissue where her clitoris had been and the front wall of her vagina. She finally was able to have an orgasm by using one hand to stroke herself over her scar and a finger of the other hand to caress her vagina. It only took two or three more weeks to teach this technique to Cal. He was delighted to feel that sex was a more mutual pleasure again.

Sex after Operations That Reconstruct the Vagina

Several pelvic cancer operations remove part of a woman's vagina, making reconstruction necessary.

Radical Cystectomy

When women have invasive bladder cancer, the surgeon usually removes not only the bladder, but also the urethra, uterus, ovaries, and at least part of the front wall of the vagina. Some surgeons use skin grafts to reconstruct the front part of the vagina, but more often they construct a new vaginal tube from the rear vaginal wall. Sometimes the surgeon sews together the two edges of the rear wall, forming a narrow vagina. Another strategy is to double over the rear wall and seam it on the left and right sides, creating a shallow vagina. Depending on the location of the tumor, surgeons may also be able to spare some of the front vaginal wall.

Most women take some time to adjust to having sex again after radical cystectomy. If the vagina has lost a good deal of size, using estrogen replacement, water-based lubricants, and even a set of vaginal dilators can be helpful (see Chapter 14). In a group of nine women whom I interviewed several years ago, all had been sexually active and orgasmic with intercourse before a radical cystectomy. After surgery, all of them found intercourse uncomfortable at first, but seven of the women eventually were able to have intercourse without pain.

Abdominoperineal Resection

Abdominoperineal resection for colon cancer in women usually includes removal of not only the colon and rectum, but also the uterus and ovaries. Sometimes, if a tumor is on the front wall of the rectum, the nearby back wall of the vagina also has to be removed. Vaginal reconstruction would then be part of surgery. Even if the vagina itself is not damaged, the loss of the rectum leaves a lack of cushioning behind the rear wall of the vagina.

The most common sexual problem after abdominoperineal resection is pain with intercourse. Pain is usually triggered by deep or vigorous thrusting and may be caused by scar tissue or adhesions or by tenderness on the rear vaginal wall. Women can often overcome the pain with extra lubrication, use of vaginal dilators to reduce conditioned muscle tension, and changing intercourse positions to minimize pressure on tender areas (see Chapter 14).

Total Pelvic Exenteration

Total pelvic exenteration is the most extensive radical pelvic surgery. In a woman, it means removing the bladder and urethra, uterus, ovaries, vagina, colon, and rectum. Many women have a vagina reconstructed at the time of surgery. Some surgeons use flaps made of inner-thigh skin and its underlying muscle and blood supply to sculpt a new vagina. Others use a piece of intestine to create a vaginal canal. Most women end up with both a urinary ostomy and a colostomy. Sometimes, however, surgeons can reconstruct an internal bladder or reconnect the anus and intestines.

Pelvic exenteration is used to treat cancer of the cervix that has reoccurred in the local area or that is too extensive to be cured by radical hysterectomy or radiation therapy. Even for a young woman, it takes a few months to recover from total pelvic exenteration. When a woman is having trouble just getting through the day and is learning to care for two ostomies, resuming sex is often not her highest priority.

If a woman has a vagina reconstructed from thigh muscle flaps, she may notice that stimulation to her vaginal walls feels as if her thighs were being stroked because the tissue's nerve supply remains attached to its original nerve network. Some women learn to get sexual pleasure from these feelings and can reach orgasm during intercourse. During lovemaking, pleasurable feelings from the breasts, clitoris, and other erotic zones may also compensate for the loss of feeling from the vagina. A vagina built from muscle flaps does not produce its own lubrication. Women are usually advised to use a good amount of water-based lubricant for intercourse and to douche with a mild vinegar and water solution to reduce vaginal odor.

Recently, forty women who had pelvic exenteration and reconstruction with muscle flaps filled out a questionnaire about their sex lives. About half resumed intercourse after their surgery, usually within the first year. Their most frequent concerns included feeling self-conscious about their ostomies and how they looked in the nude and having difficulties with vaginal dryness or discharge. Intercourse was also painful or gave little pleasure for a number of women.

Reconstructed vaginas made of intestine or skin grafts can produce some lubrication with sexual arousal and work quite well after some cancer operations. With pelvic exenteration, however, a drawback is that the vaginal canal may have little softness or stretchiness without underlying muscle tissue for cushioning. Intestine can also produce a discharge with an unpleasant odor. Again, regular douching is helpful, as is using extra lubrication for sexual activity.

Penectomy: Sex without a Penis

Penile cancer is a kind of squamous-cell skin cancer. It is rare (fewer than 1,000 new cases a year in the United States), but it is deadly if it invades into the bloodstream or lymph system of the pelvis. Cancers that have not spread beyond the top layers of skin cells can sometimes be treated with radiation therapy, but most tumors require removal of part or all of the penis for cure.

Partial penectomy removes the glans, or head of the penis, and some portion of the shaft. It is the surgery of choice, but it can only be performed if a man will be left with enough penile length to direct his stream of urine away from his body. Typically the shaft that is left can get erect with sexual arousal. A man can still reach orgasm with sexual stimulation and ejaculate through the opening at the end of the remaining penis. For many men, the shaft is long enough to penetrate a partner's vagina and thrust for intercourse, though the positions that work may be limited by the length of the erection.

Total penectomy is a more extensive operation in which the entire penis is removed along with the lymph nodes in the groin area. Plastic surgery may be needed to cover the area of the incisions with new tissue. A new opening, called a *perineal urethrostomy*, must be created for urination. The opening is placed behind the testicles but in front of the anus. The internal valve that allows a man to control the flow of his urine remains undamaged, but he must sit to urinate. Many men who have penile cancer are quite elderly and adjust to this operation by simply giving up on sex. Those who wish to remain sexually active after penectomy often find they are still able to experience sexual pleasure and reach orgasm. When they have a climax, they ejaculate semen through the perineal urethrostomy.

Some men have their first orgasm after surgery during an erotic dream. Men also learn to reach orgasm through sexual caressing of remaining sensitive genital areas, such as the scrotum, the perineal skin behind the scrotum, and the skin around the area where the penis was removed. It may take some practice to find sexual caressing that is arousing. Men may wish to use sexual fantasies, erotic videos or stories, or a vibrator to enhance their excitement. If a man wanted to father a child, his semen could be collected when he ejaculated and used to inseminate his partner.

Urinary Ostomies: Sex without a Bladder

If a person needs a radical cystectomy to treat localized bladder cancer, the surgeon needs to construct a new pathway for urine to exit the body. Most people have an ileal conduit and urinary ostomy: An opening is made in the abdomen and connected to the kidneys via a tube created out of intestine. As the kidneys make urine, it drips through the new tube and out of the ostomy, where it is collected in a plastic bag. The bag fits into a *faceplate* that is glued to the skin. The bag can be emptied a number of times a day through a valve at the bottom, but the faceplate only needs changing every few days. The ostomy appliance is watertight and does not have an odor as long as it is cared for properly.

In recent years, surgeons have also developed ways to construct an internal bladder out of intestine. One option is to have a continent ostomy: Urine does not leak out of the opening and the internal urine reservoir can be emptied every few hours by putting a soft catheter into the ostomy. The rest of the time, a dressing is worn over the ostomy, and an appliance is not needed. An even more complex operation can create a new bladder that hooks up to the urethra. The on/off valve that controls normal urination is preserved so that natural urination can occur as desired, through the same opening as always. Bladder reconstruction adds more time to the cancer surgery and increases the risk of complications. Most patients who choose these newer options are on the younger and more active side.

If you wear a urinary ostomy appliance, there are a number of ways to minimize the sexual impact. Always empty urine from the pouch before starting lovemaking to avoid a leak or odor during sex. You may want to avoid eating foods, such as asparagus, that give urine a strong scent. Some men or women get smaller pouches for their appliance to wear during sexual activity so the pouch will not get in the way as much. These pouches need to be emptied more frequently than the larger ones, of course.

Ostomy supply catalogs sell pouch covers or sewing patterns so that you can make your own covers. Women often make cloth covers out of pretty materials or even trimmed with lace to match lingerie. Men may choose comfortable terry cloth. Another way to keep the appliance out of the way during sex is to tape it down. If you wear a supporting belt on your faceplate, you can even tuck your emptied pouch into it for brief periods. Women often like to wear camisoles or panties that cover the pouch or ostomy opening. Some lingerie stores or catalogs sell panties made without a crotch so that the vulva is available for caressing.

You may think that a man would have an easier time than a woman coping with a urinary ostomy because physical attractiveness is traditionally more valued for women. In my experience, men may feel as much shame and insecurity about having an ostomy as women do. Men also have an added burden: Whereas society tends to give women a fair amount of permission to complain about an illness and to express sadness about physical changes they experience, men are expected, first, not to feel upset about a physical loss, and, second, to hide any bad feelings they do have.

Being a family man was Otis's highest priority. He and his wife, Erna, raised five kids and put them through college. Sometimes Otis worked seven days a week in the steel mills and did odd jobs on the side. He had been a minor league baseball player in his early twenties, and still liked to play sports whenever possible. People said he was a fine figure of a man, tall and very dark-skinned. Erna, a school teacher, was very proud of her husband. When he told her he had found blood in his urine, she urged him to see a doctor immediately. She had been nagging him to quit smoking for years, but Otis said that cigarettes were his way of unwinding after a long day.

He was 63 when his bladder cancer was diagnosed, and a radical cystectomy was recommended. Because cancer cells were also found in the lining of Otis's urethra, the whole urinary tube had to be removed, ruling out an internal bladder reconstruction. Otis hated his ostomy appliance. When he first got home, he persuaded Erna to change his faceplate every few days, but she finally drew the line. "What if you spring a leak when I'm at work?" Erna wanted to know. "Are you going to call me to come from school and change you? You've always been a proud man, and you need to take care of this yourself." Otis grumbled, but he got used to handling his ostomy equipment.

Resuming sex was something else again. Otis could not bear the thought of touching his wife without being able to get an erection. The fact that he had taken early retirement when his cancer was diagnosed, and now had all day to sit alone at home, did not help his mood. He became chronically depressed and gained fifteen pounds. The extra weight made his ostomy faceplate fit less well, and he kept having leaks. Although he did not express any of these thoughts to Erna, she guessed what was wrong. She had the pastor from their church come and talk to Otis, but his suggestion to be grateful to God and remember the story of Job did not comfort Otis very much. What did help in the end was his urologist's suggestion to try penile injection therapy. Being able to have erections and intercourse again boosted Otis's spirits and helped Erna, in turn, feel like her man was back.

Nerve-sparing techniques have been used in radical cystectomy for men. Recently Dr. Patrick Walsh and his colleagues at Johns Hopkins reported that after nerve-sparing radical cystectomy, 62 percent of men in their forties, 47 percent of men in their fifties, 43 percent of men in their sixties, and 20 percent of men in their seventies recovered usable erections. If the entire urethra needs to be removed as part of surgery, erections are less likely to recover. Because the prostate and seminal vesicles are gone, a man will no longer ejaculate semen, although he still can have the sensation of orgasm. Some surgeons worry that nerve-sparing cystectomy has a higher risk of leaving cancer behind.

Sex with a Colostomy or Ileostomy

Surgery to remove cancer in the colon or rectum varies in extent, depending on the size and location of the tumor. Some people end up with a colostomy or an ileostomy to eliminate stool. Others are able to have reconstructive surgery to connect the anal canal to the end of the remaining intestine. They can then eliminate stool through the anus, but they may have some leakage of stool, chronic loose stools, or urgency when they need to have a bowel movement.

If you have an ileostomy, it is active much of the time, so you need to wear an ostomy pouch continually. Pouch covers or lingerie can help camouflage the ostomy appliance during lovemaking (see previous suggestions for urinary ostomies). If you have a colostomy, you may be able to use irrigation (using a liquid solution to wash the stool out of your intestines) to regulate the times when stool comes out. If you had pelvic radiation, however, or if your bowels tended to move multiple times a day before surgery, you may not be able to irrigate successfully. Irrigation is helpful, although it is a bit time-consuming, because you can just wear a dressing, a small safety pouch, or a stoma cap over your ostomy for lovemaking. You can also plan lovemaking at times when your ostomy is least active. In general, you may want to avoid eating high-fiber foods that create gas in the hours before a planned session of lovemaking.

If you have had reconstructive bowel surgery and pass stool through your anus, you may still worry about leakage during sex. You may want to plan sex at times of day when you are less likely to have bowel movements, limit your food intake in the hours before sex, or watch the type of foods you eat. If an accident happens, both partners can jump in the shower and go back to bed afterward.

The risk that colorectal cancer surgery will damage a man's erection capacity depends on whether the nerves that run between the prostate and rectum are damaged. As with surgery to remove the prostate and bladder, nerve-sparing techniques are increasingly used when the location and size of the tumor allow. Men who are concerned about erection problems after surgery can find the information they need in Chapters 10 and 11. Some men end up with dry orgasms because of nerve damage during surgery, as discussed in Chapters 12 and 18.

Brian was a software designer in California's Silicon Valley. He and his lover, Scott, had been living together for two years when Brian was found to have rectal cancer. Although Brian and Scott felt very committed to each other, they each occasionally had other sexual partners. Both men were very careful to use condoms and other safer sex techniques. Because Brian's tumor was aggressive and very low in the rectum, his surgery was extensive and he had to have a colostomy. Scott reassured Brian over and over that he remained committed to him and had no intention of leaving, but Brian became deeply depressed.

Brian had been scrupulous about working out daily, but now he refused to go to the health club because of his shame over being seen in the locker room with his colostomy appliance. He no longer wanted to join Scott to attend concerts or hang out at their favorite coffeehouse. When friends called, he told them he was too tired to see them. His life was restricted to work and sitting in the house. For a month or two, Scott also stayed home. Eventually, however, he felt he was only catering to Brian's self-destructiveness by giving up his own social life.

When Scott came home after midnight from an evening with friends, he found Brian unconscious on their bed. Brian had taken an overdose of tranquilizers, but the paramedics were able to get him to the emergency room in time to save his life. Scott gave Brian an ultimatum that he would only stay in the relationship if they got counseling together. In the sessions, Brian expressed his fear that neither Scott nor any other man would love or want him. "I not only have this ugly, disgusting thing on my side," he said tearfully, "but I can't have anal sex anymore either." The therapist pointed out that Scott had always been the more jealous and insecure partner. Now the tables had turned. Scott reassured Brian many times that neither anal sex nor physical perfection was necessary to their relationship. He even joked that now Brian would be forced to have safer sex. He did need to know, however, that Brian would never try to hurt himself again.

Brian promised Scott that he would never make another suicide attempt. He continued with some counseling to work on coming to terms with the changes in his body and his life.

Laryngectomy: Sex without a Voice Box

We have been talking in this chapter about missing parts of the reproductive system. The *larynx*, or voice box, is not an organ we think about as sexual, but losing it does have an impact on lovemaking. When your larynx has to be removed to treat cancer, a new opening is created in your throat for breathing and speech. Some people are able to learn esophageal speech (a way of talking by using swallowed air). Others have mechanical speech aids that magnify the sounds they can produce. Speech aids make your voice sound flat and tinny, however, without the subtle tones that normally convey feelings.

The *tracheostomy*, or opening, is not pleasant to see. Mucus tends to collect around it, which has to be wiped off frequently. You can cover your tracheostomy with a scarf or high-necked shirt that is loose and light enough to allow easy breathing.

Having a tracheostomy means that communication through words may be difficult during sex. It may be awkward to speak, or the words may have to convey the whole message, without depending on tone of voice. Sweet nothings whispered with a speech aid may sound a little comical. A sense of humor definitely helps in adjusting to laryngectomy. One man told his support group that he thought he was better at kissing since his surgery. "Now I never have to come up for air," he declared. You may want to use more nonverbal communication to guide your partner during lovemaking. Your partner also has to get used to feeling your breath coming from your throat, an unexpected sensation. Whether you decide to cover your tracheostomy during sex is up to you.

Tracey had always been proud of her body. Even at age 51, she was in good enough shape to wear a bikini at the beach. She had resisted giving up smoking because of her intense fear that she would gain weight. When she had to have a laryngectomy, having the tracheostomy was even more upsetting to her than the loss of her voice. She gradually acquired a whole wardrobe of neckwear, however. For sex, she bought small chiffon scarves that she could tie around her neck. Her husband told her that they were a turn-on. "You look like one of the nudes in an old, French painting," he commented. Tracey was able to use esophageal speech, but she remained self-conscious about others' reactions to her unusual voice quality. She wished she could camouflage her speech as successfully as she hid her changed appearance. Tracey was an outgoing person, however, and found that helping others made her feel less sorry for herself. She became a central organizer in her local chapter of the United

Ostomy Association (see Resources under Information Networks) and arranged a successful fashion show as a fund raiser.

Having sex despite a missing part is one good example of courage in the face of cancer. Another group of survivors began fighting their cancer before they even had the resources of adulthood. The next chapter focuses on men and women who had cancer in childhood or adolescence and the reproductive issues they face.

26

Survivors of Childhood Cancer

Medicine has made remarkable progress in treating childhood cancers. Since 1950, the rate of death from childhood malignancies has fallen by 60 percent. Over two-thirds of all children diagnosed with cancer before age 15 are successfully treated. Thus, in the United States there are currently more than 150,000 people who have survived pediatric cancer. Yet we know very little about survivors' sex lives and fertility.

Childhood Cancer and Long-Term Health

Treatment for childhood cancers often includes chemotherapy and may also involve radiation therapy and/or surgery. Long-term effects can include learning disabilities (mainly if a child had radiation therapy to the brain), delays in reaching puberty, shortened adult height, or damage to testicles or ovaries. Some survivors may be at increased risk for second cancers; for example, girls treated for Hodgkin's disease with radiation are at risk later on for breast cancer.

We do know that survivors of pediatric cancer are somewhat less likely to marry than their peers or siblings. For those who do marry, however, divorce rates are no different than for the rest of the population.

Although adult survivors of pediatric cancer have slightly reduced fertility as a group, most are able to have children. As in older men and women, radiation directly to the testicles in boys or the use of alkylating chemotherapy drugs in boys or girls are the treatments most destructive to future fertility (see Chapters 17 and 19).

If damage is severe, a child will need hormone treatment in order to go through puberty. For teenage girls, the hormones trigger growth of breasts and body hair and cause menstruation. In boys, the hormones help the penis and testicles grow to full size and stimulate body hair, beard growth, and voice changes. Most of these teens will need to take hormones for the rest of their adult lives to maintain normal physique and sexual desire. Ironically, girls who get radiation to the skull and brain occasionally develop early puberty and are given hormones to delay physical changes and to ensure a more normal adult height.

Second Generation: Children of Childhood Cancer Survivors

Researchers have not found an increased risk of birth defects or cancer in children born to cancer survivors. In fact, out of 4,256 such children followed, only 33 developed cancer in childhood. Twenty-five of these were children who had inherited the gene for retinoblastoma, a pediatric cancer that can be inherited (although most cases of retinoblastoma are caused by environmental factors, rather than inheritance).

Although our current knowledge makes us optimistic about the health of children born to cancer survivors, if you are a woman survivor, you may want to consult an obstetrician who takes care of high-risk pregnancies, especially if cancer treatment included any radiation therapy to the pelvis or abdominal area or if you had chemotherapy with drugs such as doxorubicin or daunorubicin. It is a good idea for any childhood cancer survivor to see a geneticist if you are planning to have a baby. A few childhood cancers involve a gene mutation you could pass on. If your family is small or does not communicate, you may be unaware of patterns of cancer. Sometimes in the years after you had cancer, other members of the family also develop malignancies that suggest a genetic risk. A boy with a sarcoma of the bone, for example, may be the first person in his family known to have cancer. By the time he is 25, however, his older sister has had breast cancer and a first cousin has developed a brain tumor. This group of cancers could be caused by a flawed gene. A geneticist can either give reassurance that an inherited cancer gene is unlikely or provide information on genetic testing if a risk is pinpointed. (See Chapter 21 for a description of genetic testing for cancer risk and suggestions on how to find a genetic counseling program.)

The Emotional Impact of Surviving Childhood Cancer

The emotional impact on adults of having had cancer as a child varies widely. Your reactions may depend on the age at which your cancer occurred, how your family and medical team chose to handle it at the time, and whether the cancer had long-term effects on your health.

Secrets in the Family

Some men or women only find out about their childhood cancer as an adult. They may recall being sick as a child, but they were never been told the name of their illness. If the cancer occurred in very early childhood, they may not even remember it. Before the 1960s, cancer was seen as a stigma, and even medical professionals did not always discuss it openly. More recently, large hospitals and cancer centers have routinely provided counseling and support for children and their parents, including advice on what and when to tell the child.

Parents may feel they are doing the best for their child by hiding the trauma of cancer; but keeping it a secret is rarely helpful. For one thing, secrecy can make a child feel more stigmatized, as if the illness is so nightmarish that it cannot even be mentioned. Lack of knowledge about health history also interferes with good future health care. Openness has increasingly been encouraged.

Even if parents tell a child he or she has cancer, they may not understand or explain the possible later impact, such as the chance of infertility or other future health problems. After a number of years, childhood cancer survivors often stop seeing the cancer specialists who treated them and, thus, are at risk for being uninformed.

Chris and his wife, Dana, had been married for five years when they felt ready to start a family. After a year and a half of trying, they decided to see a doctor to find out why no pregnancy had occurred. Dana's gynecologist had her keep temperature charts for several months. They showed a picture-perfect ovulation pattern. Before having Dana go through more tests, the gynecologist asked Chris to have a semen analysis. Both partners were stunned when the results came back—no live sperm were seen. A hormone test also showed elevated FSH (follicle-stimulating hormone), suggesting Chris's testicles were not working.

"But I have three brothers, and they all have kids," Chris told the urologist. "Why should this happen to me?" The urologist asked Chris about his health history. Chris recalled being in the hospital for a quite a while during second grade, but he had no idea what had been wrong. Because Chris knew the name of the hospital, the urologist asked him to get his old health records sent over.

Two weeks later, Chris got a call from the urologist's office, asking him to make an appointment to come in. Dana wanted to come along to hear what the doctor had to say. "I have some news that may surprise you," the urologist told Chris and Dana. "The illness you had as a child was acute lymphoblastic leukemia, the most common childhood cancer."

Chris could not believe it and asked to read the record himself. The urologist showed Chris his diagnosis. He then explained that Chris's fertility problem occurred because of his cancer treatment, which included chemotherapy and radiation to the testicles. He offered to perform a testicular biopsy to see if Chris was producing any live sperm cells that could be used with new infertility treatments (see Chapter 18). The couple could also consider using semen from a donor or adopting.

After the couple went home, Chris cried for two hours. Dana hugged him and told him over and over that she still loved him and they would find a way to have a baby. Then Chris's grief turned to anger. His parents lived a few miles away, and, despite Dana's pleading to wait a few days until he had time to think everything through, Chris stormed out to his car and drove to confront them.

Chris's parents were first-generation Greek immigrants who had never gone to college. They had worked hard to give their children an education and all the advantages they had lacked themselves. They were as unprepared for their son's rage as he had been for the news of his leukemia and infertility. "We only did what we thought was best for you," his mother kept repeating.

"The doctors told us not to tell you," his father explained. "They said you were too young to understand and you would just be frightened. I don't even remember them mentioning fertility. You don't know how close you were to dying! We just were praying that you would live."

After all three family members cried together, Chris forgave his parents. He realized that they had not had any guidance at the time from the doctors on how to help him with the emotional side of leukemia. He and Dana would not have an easy time getting used to this new information, but they would cope. When they did adopt a baby girl, Chris's parents loved her just as much as their other grandchildren, and much of the family's grief was healed.

The Doomsday Syndrome

Most adult survivors are very much aware of their childhood cancer history. In fact, studies of people treated for cancer in later childhood or adolescence suggest that many are left with lingering anxieties. They worry about their health and the chance that cancer may reoccur. Some people become focused on physical symptoms, panicking if they have a minor ache or pain. When distress is strong, a young man or woman may drift aimlessly through life, having trouble investing in a relationship or career because of the feeling that there is no future. Some may rule out ever having a child, without any medical reason to think a baby would not be healthy.

Not only internal roadblocks but also external forces can limit a cancer survivor's options. Even though a cancer happened in childhood and was successfully treated, some insurance companies or employers discriminate against survivors. Because there are laws protecting against employment discrimination, the prejudice is only revealed in subtle ways—some other excuse is found to avoid hiring. The National Coalition for Cancer Survivorship (see Resources under Information Networks) provides helpful information about fighting discrimination.

Despair about the future may lead a man or woman to have casual, short-term sexual relationships, without developing deep feelings for anyone. For women who see themselves as damaged, sex without intimacy may be a way of getting some attention from men. A feeling of doom can also provide an excuse to ignore safer sex. Some survivors may avoid dating altogether, feeling that they will be rejected by potential mates.

Doris was the third out of five children fathered by three different men. Her mother was never married and was an alcoholic. Doris was 10 when she was found to have a nasopharyngeal (sinus) tumor. It was treated with radiation therapy and chemotherapy. Because of the radiation, one side of Doris's facial bones did not grow normally. Her eyes were not level with each other, and one was larger. One cheekbone was not symmetrical and Doris's mouth was drawn into a sneer. She had lost several teeth, although she was able to wear dentures to compensate. Her voice was mildly slurred.

By the time she was a young woman, Doris was chronically depressed. She had become quite overweight and took little care with her appearance. One of her mother's many boyfriends had introduced Doris to sex at age 12. Although she found his attentions painful and sometimes disgusting, she craved the small treats and affectionate gestures she got after being molested. She ran away from home at 15 and was pregnant at 16. Doris's two children were the center of her life, but she had no job skills to earn enough to support them. She lived on welfare and, following in her mother's footsteps, had a series of violent, alcohol-abusing partners.

Doris finally got some help after her own daughter told her that one of the boyfriends had tried to rape her. Doris not only broke up with the man, but started family therapy with her children. The therapist helped Doris find a job-skills training program, and she became a child care worker. Eventually she married a stable, older man who was loving to her and the children.

Body Image Issues

Although some survivors must live with physical changes, such as an amputated limb or an ostomy, the fact that they have experienced the difficulty since childhood has allowed them to build good coping skills. To an outsider, they seem extremely brave, but internally they just feel normal. They become a one-legged skier or an aerobics teacher with a colostomy. They also begin their sexual lives knowing that their bodies are different and that partners will have to value them as they are.

> When Stephanie had her urostomy for a rhabdomyosarcoma of the bladder, she was only 4 years old. The enterostomal therapist taught her how to change her appliance by having her practice with a toy one on her rag doll. Petite, blond Stephanie never let her outside bladder stop her from doing what she wanted, whether it was ice-skating lessons or cheerleading squad.
>
> Stephanie knew she could never have children because her surgery had also removed her uterus. As she grew older, she had no lack of boyfriends, however. Stephanie's experiences with illness as a child decided her on a career as a pediatrician. She graduated from medical school at the top of her class. During her residency, she married her steady boyfriend from college, an architect.
>
> She sent her enterostomal therapist letters every year, including pictures from her wedding and honeymoon. The nurse kept Stephanie's pictures on a bulletin board in her office, and the beautiful bride in the photograph comforted many young girls who were going to have to have an ostomy.

As I write this chapter, the National Cancer Institute has just added a special program, the Office of Cancer Survivorship, to study the long-term problems and needs of cancer survivors. It is hoped that the children who are being treated for cancer today will benefit from increased knowledge about preventing and treating sexual problems and infertility related to childhood cancer.

27

Gay and Lesbian Cancer Survivors

Almost all of the information in this book is relevant to gay men and women with cancer. Men and women who have lovers of the same sex do not differ in any major physical way from heterosexuals. Their genital and pelvic organs and hormone systems are normal. They also share the same concerns of other men and women about the impact of cancer on attractiveness and desirability in romantic and sexual relationships. This chapter highlights a few issues, however, that are uniquely important to gay men and women facing cancer.

Sexual Orientation and Your Cancer Risk

In the United States, recent estimates are that about 4 percent of men and about 2 percent of women have mainly homosexual relationships. A much larger group of Americans has occasional sexual experiences with the same sex. Assuming that gay and heterosexual people have the same risk of cancer, at least 27,000 gay men and 11,500 gay women had new cancer diagnoses in 1995, based on the American Cancer Society's national statistics. This is a large group of people whose needs are usually ignored.

In fact, both gay men and women may be at increased risk for certain types of cancer, but for very different reasons. Most gay men have steady relationships with one or a few men, but others have casual sex with many different partners. In the 1970s and 1980s, gay communities in urban centers fostered a new pride and openness. Part of this movement was a call to enjoy sexual freedom. Men who experimented with many partners

226

were vulnerable to sexually transmitted diseases (STDs). Because gay communities are relatively small, it was easy for viruses like the human immunodeficiency virus (HIV), hepatitis B, or the human papilloma virus (HPV) to spread within them. Each of these viruses may promote a few types of cancer.

The stigma of the AIDS epidemic adds to the burden of gay men who develop cancer. Some men may indeed be positive for HIV. Their damaged immune systems cannot fight cancer effectively. They are also more prone to infections and other life-threatening complications of cancer treatment. Men who are HIV-negative still may be stigmatized by people who assume the cancer is a symptom of a fatal case of AIDS or, at least, is related in some way to homosexuality. Most special resources for gay men with cancer are found as part of organizations that help men with AIDS (see Resources under Information Networks).

Gay women, in contrast, are the group in our society with the lowest rate of STDs. Surveys suggest that gay women typically have exclusive live-in partnerships, although they may experience several such relationships over the years. Gay women's cancer risk may be higher for breast or ovarian cancer, however, because of their reproductive histories. These malignancies are more common in women who do not have children or who experience their first pregnancy later in life. Many lesbian women never get pregnant or, if they do choose to be a mother, wait until their thirties when they are more financially secure. Some lesbians not only have increased cancer risk, but also neglect to have annual cancer screening, including pap smears and mammograms. Because women in general earn less than men, some gay women cannot afford good health care. Others believe that they are not at risk for reproductive system cancers because they are lesbians, or they avoid seeing a doctor after experiencing prejudice in health care settings because of their sexual orientation. Lesbians should be aware of a very helpful resource, The Mary-Helen Mautner Project for Lesbians with Cancer (see Resources under Information Networks).

Being Gay in the Health Care System

Unfortunately, health care professionals in the United States are often homophobic and ignorant about gay lifestyles. If you are open about your lifestyle, you may run into overt prejudice, such as having a doctor or nurse wear rubber gloves in a situation where it is not necessary. More subtle discrimination may take the form of cold and disapproving looks from medical staff or the physician's not offering a pap smear because he or she thinks that lesbians do not get cervical cancer. On top of all the other stresses of having cancer, you do not need a hostile health care environment.

What can you do to avoid discrimination?

- As much as your insurance plan allows, use your network of friends and colleagues to find physicians who are positive about gay lifestyles. This is especially helpful if your cancer treatment has caused a sexual problem.

- Be assertive if you feel your health care provider is homophobic. First try dignified confrontation; for example, "I feel you are uncomfortable discussing my health with me because I am gay, but I need my questions answered." If nothing changes, ask for a different doctor or nurse. If you are part of a managed care plan that does not want to provide an alternate referral, make a formal complaint about the discrimination. Keep a diary of events with dates, names, observations, and quotes. Tell your provider that you are tape-recording your visits so that you will remember medical information accurately.

One special form of discrimination is legally sanctioned. Because gay relationships do not have the status of marriages, your lover may not be given the normal rights of a spouse to visit, participate in sessions with the doctor, have access to crucial medical information, or make decisions about your health care if you are very ill. Even if you informally designate your lover as the one responsible for health care decisions in an emergency, your parents or other family members can interfere and make trouble. Therefore, it is important to have legal forms that are signed and entered in your medical record and to give copies of the forms to your partner. Because these issues arise so often for men with AIDS, gay organizations offer counseling and legal advice on giving a partner health or financial power of attorney.

A gay couple also may not receive the same support as a heterosexual couple outside of the medical system. In the workplace, it is rare that a company will recognize a gay relationship in providing benefits such as family leave to care for an ill partner. If you are not open about your relationship, not only coworkers but other important people in your partner's life may not realize the trauma that he or she is experiencing as a caretaker. Even when both sides of the family know about the relationship, they may not always give you the practical help or emotional support you need.

If you do not have a committed partner, you may find yourself in an even lonelier situation than a single heterosexual person, especially if your relationships with family members are strained or if you moved away from family to live in a place with a larger gay community. Although there are many support groups and volunteer organizations to help people with AIDS and people with cancer, HIV-negative gay people with cancer may feel that they will not be accepted or understood in either setting. If you are in this situation, it may be up to you to be creative and reach out to your friends or to take a risk and try getting support from places that were not designed with your particular lifestyle in mind. Mental health professionals who are comfortable with homosexuality can also provide emotional support in individual counseling.

Gay Sexuality after Cancer

Because gay sexual relationships are not structured by marriage, you have the advantage of flexibility. Both gay men and women tend to have more variety in their sex lives than heterosexual couples. Your imaginations are not constrained by the traditional model of sex we all learn through our culture—kissing, a little foreplay, penis-in-vagina intercourse, and off to sleep. Gay sex may include kissing, caressing, oral sex, anal stimulation, or penetration of the vagina or anus with a partner's fingers or with a penis-shaped sex toy. Other variations, such as dominance/submission games or group sex, are common in some networks of gay people just as they are among some heterosexuals.

Having a varied sex life is a great help in coping with changes in sexual function after cancer treatment. A lesbian woman who developed pain with vaginal penetration after radiation therapy could still enjoy all sorts of breast and clitoral caressing and might be less distressed than a heterosexual woman whose experiences had focused on intercourse. A gay man with an erection problem could still enjoy giving and receiving oral and manual stimulation.

The focus on erotic skill in gay sex may also increase the impact of losing sexual function, however. Many gay men do seek help for an erection problem because having a hard penis is a central turn-on to themselves and their partners, whether or not they penetrate another man during lovemaking. A gay man may also be more distressed than a heterosexual man about having dry orgasms because ejaculating during hand or oral stimulation is more common between men. Gay men typically find semen more sexually arousing than heterosexual women do, so dry orgasms would be more of a loss to the partner. For gay women, oral sex is often an important, shared pleasure. Radical vulvectomy would feel especially mutilating to a gay woman who has more comfort than the average heterosexual woman with her own genitals and expects her partner to be aroused by seeing, touching, and tasting them.

Gay men and women may find some inspiration in books or videos about gay sexuality. Some of the techniques suggested to enhance pleasure may also help couples to overcome a sexual problem related to cancer treatment. Most urban areas have a gay or feminist bookstore that carries such materials. Another good source is The Sexuality Library catalog (see Resources under Products to Enhance Sex).

Cliff was diagnosed with prostate cancer when he was 62. He and his longtime lover Joshua were both social workers, but Joshua was in his early forties. Cliff was relieved that his cancer was localized, but he was very worried about the impact of his radical prostatectomy on his relationship. He and Joshua each occasionally had other casual partners, but their sex life together had remained exciting and special. Jealousy was rarely an issue because their lives were so intertwined and they were the best of friends as well as sexual partners.

Joshua told Cliff that he would not stop loving him, even if he never had another erection. He also minimized his feelings about Cliff losing the ability to ejaculate semen. Both men, however, were saddened by trying to have sex without an erection. Even though Cliff still had orgasms, reaching them took much longer, and he could see that Joshua lost much of his excitement before that point. When the two of them went out with friends, Cliff found himself watching Joshua's reactions to other men and feeling insecure.

Cliff's urologist did not seem aware of his sexual orientation. He did give Cliff some information about sex after prostatectomy, but all the booklets assumed that the man was heterosexual. Cliff decided to continue playing the game, just to make life easier. At his one-year follow-up, he mentioned that he had not noticed any return of firm erections, either on waking from sleep or with his partner. The urologist agreed with Cliff's request to have a penile prosthesis implanted.

Cliff and Joshua made many jokes about Cliff's new, bionic penis. They even told their closest friends about the operation. "I don't want it getting around town too much," Joshua teased Cliff, "or else I'm afraid you'll be out every night giving demonstrations." Cliff had no intention of using his prosthesis to try out a string of new partners, but it felt good to hear Joshua expressing some envy, instead of vice versa.

Standards of Beauty and Physical Changes from Cancer

Gay men's erotica is often very focused on physical beauty, whereas lesbian women's sexual images are less apt to show conventional feminine prettiness. Surveys of same-sex couples suggest that life, at least to some extent, imitates art. In their study of committed relationships published in the book *American Couples* (see Resources under Books), sociologists Pepper Schwartz and Philip Blumstein found that only lesbian couples disregarded the power of physical attractiveness. Gay male and heterosexual couples were very aware of the role of beauty in their sexual attraction.

The physical disfigurement caused by some cancer treatments may be particularly difficult for a gay man, especially because our society gives women a good deal of sympathy and support if they lose a breast or experience baldness but expects men to tough it out, baring their scars nonchalantly or wearing a baseball cap rather than a wig.

Lesbian women also care about how they look and are likely to feel as much sadness as any woman about losing a breast or experiencing other physical changes from cancer therapy. If a woman is part of a social network of other gay women, however, she often will have a strong emotional support system of friends who do not feel obligated to live up to the images in the heterosexual world of women's fashion magazines and TV shows.

> When Terry went through chemotherapy, she decided not to wait for her hair to fall out in clumps like the other women at the hospital. Instead, she asked her lover, Brooke, to shave her head. Terry was quite tall and liked to wear bold, dangling earrings and pants outfits in ethnic prints. At the design studio where she worked, everyone admired her new look. Sometimes she varied it by wearing African or Peruvian caps. She became so comfortable with the unique style that she decided to continue to shave her head, even after her chemotherapy was finished.

Infertility Matters to Gay People, Too

Being gay does not necessarily mean forgoing parenthood. Some gay men or women were previously in heterosexual relationships and had children before entering a gay lifestyle. Others continue to be bisexual. Gay men sometimes adopt a child, or a very few have had a child with a surrogate mother. Lesbian women often use insemination from a friend or anonymous donor to conceive. Before AIDS became an issue, it was becoming more common for a gay man and lesbian woman to join forces to have a child together through insemination with the father's sperm. Laura Benkov, in her excellent book *Reinventing the Family: The Emerging Story of Lesbian and Gay Parents* (see Resources under Books), sees a resurgence of these co-parenting arrangements with the advent of HIV testing.

For gay men or women who had planned to have a biological child and had their dreams interrupted by cancer treatment, the information in Part III of this book is all relevant. Not every infertility program will work with a gay person or couple, however. Many have a policy that they will only help married, heterosexual couples. Although such rules could certainly be challenged in court, an easier solution in most big cities is to find the infertility clinics willing to help gay people. If a woman still has normal ovulation and a healthy uterus, another option for her is to obtain semen by mail order from a commercial sperm bank and to inseminate herself at home. (See Bibliography for Chapter 27 for books and articles on this subject.)

Opal had Hodgkin's disease in her early twenties. She never seriously considered having a child until she was 32 and she and her lover, Yvonne, had been living together for three years. Neither woman had ever been pregnant. Yvonne worked long hours as a nurse in an intensive care unit, whereas Opal had a less physically demanding job as a kindergarten teacher. With Opal's love for little children, it seemed natural for her to be the partner who had a child, although Yvonne did not rule out the possibility that she, too, would have a baby in a few more years.

As the couple considered their options, the picture changed, however. Opal's menstrual cycles were irregular, and an FSH test showed that her ovaries had been damaged by her cancer treatment. If she were to have donor insemination, her gynecologist felt she should also take hormones. Even then, it was unclear if Opal could become pregnant. Because she had also had radiation therapy to her abdomen, Opal would have a high-risk pregnancy and might deliver prematurely. The final straw was that Opal's principal at school did not know about her sexual orientation and had reacted very negatively when another of the unmarried teachers in the school had a baby. Opal was worried that he would find a way to fire her if she, too, became pregnant.

The two women reconsidered and decided that Yvonne would try for a pregnancy instead of Opal. They planned to spend the rest of their lives together and wanted to have a family of their own. It was worth it to Yvonne to find a less demanding nursing job that would give her more time and energy to be a parent. She moved to a home health care agency and also entered a donor insemination program. When her son Julian was born, Yvonne and Opal shared all of the parenting tasks except breast-feeding. Opal still had times of feeling sad and left out, but she felt that nurturing Julian and her children at school fulfilled many of her needs.

Gay men have fewer options for being a biological parent, unless they are lucky enough to be able to afford a surrogate or to have a female friend willing to have a child with or for them.

Some states now have laws allowing gay men and women to become adoptive or foster parents. These issues are thoroughly discussed in Laura Benkov's book mentioned earlier. Benkov also wrote about the tragedies that can happen when a gay parent dies without giving legal guardian status to the person he or she would choose to raise a child. A gay parent who has had cancer should make sure to consult an attorney and make the best legal arrangements possible. Otherwise, a lover who has been the child's second emotional parent not only may lose custody, but also may end up with no contact or power to intervene in that child's life.

We should know a lot more than we do about the impact of cancer on the sexual lives and reproductive plans of gay men and women. Research is just beginning to tackle these important topics, but it is still much easier to get government funding to study how to stop people from having unsafe sex than to find out how to foster healthy sex lives in gay people after cancer. As in other areas of health, the gay community will have to continue to lobby to get its needs met.

28

Sex and the Single Survivor

Cancer survivors who are not married or in a committed relationship face some unique stresses. This chapter suggests how they can cope.

Cancer and Your Social Network

Not every single person wants to marry or even to date. Many men and women live very happy lives without a spouse or lover. A significant other is a definite asset during an illness, however. A loving spouse or partner offers practical support, such as cooking meals, providing transportation, or taking care of the kids, as well as the emotional comfort of having someone always on your side.

Unmarried people, in general, tend to have poorer health and even to die at younger ages than married people. Single men are especially likely to have poor health as compared to their married peers. Partners in a couple often encourage each other in more healthful living—cutting down on smoking and alcohol use or trying to eat more healthful foods and get more exercise. A spouse also becomes your cheerleader and chauffeur during cancer treatment.

If you are single during cancer treatment, make a list of people important to you. Some would be willing to help with concrete needs, like visiting you in the hospital, taking care of your child or pet, watering your plants, cleaning your house, driving you to doctor's appointments, or loaning you money. This list probably overlaps with the group of people in your life who can give you a listening ear, a shoulder on which to cry, some tender lovemaking, or an evening of fun that helps you forget about your illness. Try not to lean on the same one or two friends or family members for all your needs, but instead spread your requests around.

Single parents have an especially uphill battle. A recent study of single mothers with breast cancer found that they were more depressed than a similar group of married women. Single women often depended on their children for emotional support, yet the children themselves were having more difficulty coping with their mother's illness than children in two-parent families. The researchers concluded that these mothers badly needed extra support in their environments.

Support groups are a very good option for single cancer survivors. Groups introduce you to others coping with a similar health crisis and provide an atmosphere of warmth and sharing of feelings. Some research even suggests that men or women who attend groups survive longer after cancer treatment. Perhaps your local hospital or American Cancer Society has a group that would fit your needs. If you are not a "group" person, consider other activities, such as volunteer work or joining a religious congregation that might help you make some new friends and feel less alone.

Finding a Dating Partner

If you are reading this chapter, chances are you do want some type of romantic companionship. Whether you are looking for someone to date for fun or a partner for the rest of your life, you may see your cancer as an obstacle. The biggest stumbling block to finding a new partner after cancer, however, is failure to go out and look. Do not let the fear of rejection discourage you from socializing. Unless the Avon lady or a political pollster comes to your door and falls in love with you, you are unlikely to meet a new mate at home.

Research confirms that people tend to choose mates who are similar to them. People who date and marry often live very close together. They tend to be alike in age, education, religion, and ethnicity. There is even good evidence that people tend to choose partners similar to them in physical attractiveness and mental health!

Perhaps you are lucky enough to be a student or to work with a large group of single people close to you in age. Most people are outnumbered in their environments by those who are paired off, however. In the age of HIV, the singles bars and casual sex of the past two decades have lost some appeal. Still, there are ways to meet someone to date. Here are some of the more effective strategies:

- Let all of your friends know you are looking, and ask them to fix you up on some blind dates. If you dread the chance of having a boring evening, you can combine the date with some group activity that you would enjoy, such as going to a concert or having a potluck picnic.

- Try some activities that would bring you into contact with people. Choose something you would enjoy or value for its own sake so that you do not feel cheated if no friendships result. Volunteering for a charitable or political organization is one option. You may even want to get involved in a group that helps people with cancer. If your community offers some adult education classes, pick one that interests you— portrait photography, ethnic cooking, or creative writing, for example. Others in your class may become new friends or dating partners. Sports activities, such as working out in a health club, playing in a neighborhood tennis or basketball league, or coaching kids, are good ways to meet new people.

- Take advantage of resources for singles. Although singles events are often stereotyped as being only for losers, in our impersonal society they are often quite useful. Many single parents have found people to date at local Parents without Partners chapters. In large cities, newspapers or local magazines often have singles ads. Read through them each week, and consider composing one yourself. You do not have to meet anyone face to face unless you choose, and then you can control the situation by arranging to meet them in a safe, public place. Some singles organizations match you with compatible people, either through computer files or personal interviews. Singles clubs often center around a hobby, such as sailing, tennis, skiing, or hiking. Others bring together people who share the same religion.

If you have trouble approaching strangers at a social event, set yourself small goals. Instead of expecting to find your next true love, promise yourself to smile at two new people or to say hello to at least one person who might be interesting. If you attend a dance, promise yourself you will ask at least three people to dance with you. If you fulfill your goal, pat yourself on the back, even if you did not meet anybody interesting. Each time you go somewhere, give yourself a slightly more ambitious goal. Develop some skill at small talk. Read magazines or books for ideas on conversational topics. If you are really stymied, ask a friend or family member to practice with you. If you have some single friends, attending a social event with them can provide moral support.

Don't Let Your Cancer Be the Skeleton in Your Closet!

Each of us has a skeleton, yet we tend not to think about it. Seeing one, we are startled and frightened at the reminder that we will die someday. One-third of Americans will have cancer during their lifetimes. Yet cancer, especially for single people, often becomes the skeleton in the closet of our flesh—a commonplace secret that feels too horrifying to reveal.

A number of fears make it difficult to tell a potential mate about cancer. Most obvious is the fear that the cancer will return, causing disability and ultimately death. You may not worry often about your cancer history in a casual relationship, but if things get serious you may wonder whether your desirable qualities can outweigh the risk a new partner takes in making a commitment to you.

If you are interested in a lasting relationship, at some point you will want to tell your partner about your history of cancer.

Timing

Timing is a delicate issue. If you wait too long, your partner may feel a sense of betrayal that you withheld something important about yourself. It is especially important to discuss your cancer before you and your partner make important decisions, like moving in together or getting married. If you have visible scars from your cancer or a sexual problem, it is also better to reveal that information before the day you first take your clothes off together.

On the other hand, some cancer survivors are so worried about rejection that they blurt out their health history in the first few minutes to any potential mate they encounter. Even if you have many attractive qualities, you may scare away new partners if you present your illness as the central fact of your life. Once someone has had a chance to begin to know you as a friend, he or she will be more likely to accept your cancer history as part of the baggage that we all bring with us to a new relationship.

The best strategy is usually to wait to discuss your cancer until you feel that friendship and attraction are developing between the two of you. Because of concerns about HIV, many couples really take time to get to know each other these days before jumping into bed (see Chapter 6).

Getting the Words Out

It can be very anxiety provoking to imagine telling an attractive date that you have had cancer. If you have never had such a conversation, maybe a friend or family member would be willing to role-play with you. If you have no idea how to begin, try taking the role of your date, and ask your friend to play your part. Listen to your friend's words, and imagine how you would react if you were the date. Perhaps you like the way they tell the story, or maybe their communication hits you the wrong way, giving you some other ideas about what you would like to say. Once you feel more prepared, rehearse your speech with your friend as the audience. Ask your friend for feedback on how you came across.

What are the important points you want to convey? You probably do not want to be pitied as a cancer victim. Rather you want to come across as a survivor—someone who faced cancer and remains a valuable and lovable person. What is important for your partner to know about your cancer? Do you want to talk about your risk of having a recurrence? Maybe that is information you would rather not disclose unless it is a very serious relationship. Scars, ostomies, or sexual problems are important to reveal before getting sexual with someone new. Infertility or a genetic cancer risk in your family may also become an issue as a relationship develops.

The Setting

When it is time for the real thing, choose a place that you find comfortable. Many people prefer to discuss emotional topics in a private place; but if you are worried that you will cry or that your partner will get angry, a busy public place may feel safer. Avoid occasions when it would be jarring to talk about your cancer, for example, in the middle of a sexual encounter or at a holiday party.

Disclosing a Problem That Affects Your Sex Life

When cancer treatment damages your sexual function, revealing the problem in dating relationships can make a man or a woman very anxious. Women who have had a vulvectomy or vaginal reconstruction worry about how to explain their new anatomy to a partner (especially given that many men are not all that familiar with the normal arrangement of female private parts). Men who end up with erection problems may refuse to date at all until they receive treatment; and even then, they are reluctant to let a partner know they have a penile prosthesis or are using penile injections.

Glenn's prostate cancer was discovered while his wife of many years was in her final battle with breast cancer. He had a radical prostatectomy, but he really did not take much time to think about his own situation. Three months after his surgery, his wife passed away. A year later, Glenn had made many decisions in his life. He had sold his house and bought a condo in a retirement community in Arizona. There he found himself surrounded by lonely, single women. Casual dating was not Glenn's style. He was a one-woman man and wanted to remarry. He felt he could not get involved with anyone, however, until he fixed the erection problem that his surgery had left. He consulted a urologist and learned how to use penile injections (see Chapter 11).

There was a lady, Pam, who had caught Glenn's eye, and the two soon began to spend almost every day together. Pam had been widowed for ten years and had never dated anyone seriously since her husband's death. When she and Glenn finally began to kiss and touch each other, Pam was amazed to find how passionate she felt. Glenn was a considerate and skillful partner, and soon Pam felt ready to go into the bedroom. Just when she thought Glenn would suggest it, however, he stopped and said he needed to tell her something.

"What is it?" asked Pam, disappointed and worried about what Glenn might have been concealing. Glenn explained that he had had surgery for prostate cancer and no longer could get firm erections. He said he had medication to overcome the problem, but he had to give it to himself in a shot. This idea did not worry Pam, but she was taken aback when Glenn told her that the needle went into his penis. She was worried that the injection must be very painful. Glenn said that the shot did not hurt much at all. Pam said she would rather not see Glenn give himself the shot, but otherwise she thought they should pick up where they left off.

Particularly for younger people, disfigurement from cancer may be the greatest worry in dating.

Zach was only 15 when osteosarcoma was found in his leg bone. A few years earlier, he might have had to have his leg amputated, but by the time he was diagnosed, his doctors were able to use surgery, radiation, and chemotherapy to save his leg while getting rid of the tumor. Still, Zach could no longer be on the track team at school, and he went through a year of baldness from his chemotherapy. His friends all rallied around him; but his high school was big, and he often received stares from kids who did not know why one of their peers was pale, bald, and limping. Zach had always been a little shy and had not really begun to date before his illness. He would have missed his junior prom if one of the girls from his English class had not asked him to go. He worried that she had only chosen him out of pity, but he took her up on the offer anyway. Their first date was followed by others, and they eventually established a loving relationship.

Although the young couple progressed from kissing to caressing each other under their clothing, Zach did not want his girlfriend to see him with his pants off. It was only when the couple had been having intercourse for several months that Zach allowed his girlfriend to see his leg. Her acceptance was a major step in restoring his self-confidence.

Whether the issue is a change in appearance or a change in sexual capacity, you can work things out with a supportive sexual partner. If you are unsure how to get started with sexual activity, the best policy is usually to take things gradually. Try some of the suggestions in Chapter 5: Instead of expecting to have intercourse right away, start out by caressing and kissing on the couch or by exchanging back rubs. When you take more clothes off, you may feel most comfortable with very dim lighting at first. Just having sex the first time with a new partner after cancer treatment can reassure you that you are still lovable and capable of erotic pleasure.

Making a Commitment despite Infertility

One other issue that can impact on developing relationships is infertility. If you or your partner want to have children, changes in fertility related to your cancer need to be discussed openly before you make a commitment to each other. Of course many men and women who have not had cancer have to cope with infertility. Some may even have deliberately had a vasectomy or tubal ligation, only to get divorced and meet a new, childless partner who wants to start a family. Infertility on top of cancer, however, is an added threat to a dating relationship.

Sally barely remembered her bone marrow transplant. She had only been 7 years old when it happened. The isolation room and the sickness were a dim chapter in her early life. She thought she had left it all behind her until, at age 14, she had not yet developed breasts or gotten her period. Then her mother took her to the pediatrician, who explained that the cancer treatment had damaged Sally's ovaries but that he could put her on hormones so that she would go through puberty like all the other girls. He also explained that she would be unable to have a baby, although she would make a wonderful adoptive mother when she met the right man. Sally was satisfied for several years as her body developed, and she focused on the normal dramas of teenage life.

After college, Sally eventually did meet the right man. She told her boyfriend, Kyle, about her illness as a child and about her infertility. By that time, egg donation had become more common, and Sally knew that was also an option she could consider. Kyle wanted to get married, no matter what. He invited Sally to meet his family over the winter holidays. Kyle's parents gave Sally a warm welcome, although she thought they asked a few too many questions about her father's job and whether Sally planned to give up her own career in publishing after she settled down and had children.

"Have you told them about my leukemia?" she asked Kyle later that night when they were alone. Kyle said he had not. Sally was uncomfortable keeping it a secret, however, and he said he would talk to his parents before bedtime.

The next morning, it seemed to Sally that a chill had settled on the breakfast table. Kyle's father greeted her distantly, and when she sat down, his mother abruptly got up and left the table. She came back several minutes later, with reddened eyes. After the meal, Sally suggested that she and Kyle sit down with his parents and talk. As she had dreaded, they opposed the marriage strongly. They had always looked forward to having grandchildren, and Kyle was their only son. What dismayed Sally the most, however, was Kyle's reaction. He slumped silently on the couch, looking miserable. It was left to Sally to respond.

"I think I'll go upstairs and pack," she said quietly. "Kyle, could you please call a taxi to take me to the airport?"

In later years, Sally remembered this scene with pain but also with some humor. Her strongest feeling was of relief that she had called off her engagement. Kyle's immaturity and inability to stand up to his parents had truly shocked Sally. And what in-laws she would have had!

Dealing with Rejection

Fear of rejection may keep you locked into an unsatisfying relationship and prevent you from actively trying to find someone to love. Having cancer can make even a self-confident person feel insecure. How can you cope with these feelings and not allow them to isolate you?

One strategy is to imagine the worst. Suppose that you are very attracted to a new partner and that your feelings seem to be reciprocated. Then you tell him or her about your cancer, and the relationship cools. You have already had the strength to face cancer treatment. Are you going to die because someone you liked was unwilling to take the risk of getting involved with you? If this disaster happened, what would you still value in your life? What could you do to mend your hurt feelings?

Judy had been a divorced parent since her early thirties. By the time she was 50, her children were in college, and she had more free time to meet men and date. Because she was an active person who enjoyed tennis, skiing, and bridge, she had a wide circle of friends. It was not so easy, however, to find men who met her standards. When friends introduced her to William, she was really excited. He shared so many of her interests and seemed genuinely nice. He called her several times a week instead of playing hard to get, like so many of the guys she dated. When Judy told William about her colon cancer and ileostomy, he was warm and supportive, saying how he admired her strength in getting through her illness without a husband and in raising her children so successfully. Over the next two weeks, however, his phone calls were less frequent and he was always too busy to get together. Then he told Judy he was being called out of town on a prolonged business trip and would contact her when he returned. She was suspicious about this story, so it was not a total surprise to see him at the movies with another woman. Still, it made Judy feel angry and disillusioned. She decided to stop trying to date and, instead, to focus on enjoying her family, friends, and hobbies. Gradually, the pain of William's rejection lessened. The next spring, Judy met a new man quite unexpectedly and began a very satisfying relationship.

In my experience, it is more common for men to reject a woman because of her history of cancer than the reverse. Women are more comfortable with the idea of having to take care of a partner who is not in the best of health, especially because they tend to marry older mates. Of course there are exceptions to this rule. Some men are not afraid of illness and even enjoy being the white knight who rescues the needy damsel. A woman who has spent part of her life taking care of an ill husband, child, or elderly parent may want to avoid another burden at all costs. You cannot protect yourself from rejection because of a partner's fear of your illness, but you can recognize that such a breakup says more about your partner's limitations than about yours.

Some dating partners will reject you because of a physical imperfection. If you encounter one of them, it does not matter whether you have lost a leg or breast to cancer, have an ostomy, or have a more common failing, such as being overweight or having the wrong nose shape or hair color. If someone rejects you because cancer has changed your appearance, consider yourself *lucky*! Would you have wanted to get deeply involved with such a shallow person? What if you did become ill again or went through some other crisis? Would that partner stand by you? And how would that partner deal with the physical changes that aging or ill health bring to all of us?

Although it is tempting to blame failed dating relationships on your cancer, think about other factors that may have interfered. Maybe you and your partner had different politics or life goals. Perhaps you were not on the same sexual wavelength. Your personalities also may not have matched. Half of all marriages end in divorce, and a much larger percentage of dating relationships break up. You can have a happy life without a partner. If you are going to put your energy into a relationship, your mate should be someone who loves you regardless of your health.

A Final Thought

I hope this book has answered your questions and given you some resources to solve sexual difficulties or make choices about having a child. Medical knowledge is always increasing. By the time you read this book, some of the information it presents will undoubtedly be out of date. I hope you will be able to get the latest and best treatment available, however, by following the suggestions in this book on finding help. Most of all, I hope you have the quality of life you desire—including a healthy sex life and children to love.

Resources

BOOKS

Angell, M. *Science on Trial: The Clash of Medical Evidence and the Law in the Breast Implant Case*. New York: W. W. Norton & Co., 1996. Reviews the controversy over silicone breast implants.

Benkov, L. *Reinventing the Family: The Emerging Story of Lesbian and Gay Parents*. New York: Crown Publishers, 1994.

Blank, J. *Femalia*. San Francisco: Down There Press, 1993. Photos showing the variety of vulvas. (Available from the Sexuality Library.)

Blank, J. *Good Vibrations: The Complete Guide to Vibrators*. San Francisco: Down There Press, 1989. (Available from the Sexuality Library.)

Dackman, L. *Up Front: Sex and the Post-Mastectomy Woman*. New York: Penguin Books, 1990.

Gilman, L. *The Adoption Resource Book* (3d ed.). New York: HarperCollins, 1992. A comprehensive guide to adoption.

Gordon, E. *Mommy, Did I Grow in Your Tummy?* Santa Monica, CA: E. M. Greenberg Press, 1992. (Available from publisher, 1460 Seventh St., Suite 301, Santa Monica, CA 90401.) For young children, reviews several different types of assisted conception, including sperm and egg donation.

Greenwood, S. *Menopause Naturally: Preparing for the Second Half of Life*. San Francisco: Inland Books, 1992.

Hoffman, B., ed. *A Cancer Survivor's Almanac: Charting Your Journey*. Silver Spring, MD: National Coalition for Cancer Survivorship, 1996. Resources on adoption, medical care, insurance, and advocacy.

How I Began. About sperm donation; written in Australia for school-aged children. (Available from national office of Resolve, 1310 Broadway, Somerville, MA 02144-1731.)

Institute for the Advanced Study of Human Sexuality. *The Complete Guide to Safer Sex*. San Francisco: Author, 1992. (Available from the Sexuality Library.)

Ito, D. *Without Estrogen: Natural Remedies for Menopause and Beyond*. New York: Carol Southern Books, 1994.

Martin, C. *Beating the Adoption Game*. New York: Harcourt Brace Jovanovich, Publishers, 1988. A guide to adoption, including some information for cancer survivors.

Murphy, G. P., Morris, L. B., and Lange, D. (eds.). *Informed Decisions: The Complete Book of Cancer Diagnosis, Treatment, and Recovery*. New York: Viking

Penguin Books, 1997. The American Cancer Society's complete guide to cancer and its aftermath.

My Story. English book about sperm donation; aimed at very young children. (Available from Kris Probasco, ACSW, 144 Westwoods Drive, Liberty, MO 64068.)

Nessim, S., and Ellis, J. *Cancervive: The Challenge of Life after Cancer.* New York: Houghton Mifflin Co., 1991. Includes a chapter on adoption.

Schaffer, P. *How Babies and Families Are Made.* Berkeley, CA: Tabor Sarah Books, 1988. Discusses for young children a variety of ways that families come about, including semen donation, in vitro fertilization, and adoption. (Available from publisher, 2419 Jefferson, Berkeley, CA 94703.)

Schnitter, J. *Let Me Explain: A Story about Donor Insemination.* Indianapolis, IN: Perspectives Press, 1995. A book for children aged seven to ten born through donor insemination.

Schwartz, P., and Blumstein, P. *American Couples: Money, Work, Sex.* New York: Pocket Books, 1983. Surveys heterosexual and gay couples.

Zilbergeld, B. *The New Male Sexuality.* New York: Bantam Books, 1992. Self-help programs to overcome premature ejaculation and anxiety-based erection problems.

AUDIOTAPES

Zilbergeld, B., and Barbach, L. *How to Talk with a Partner about Smart Sex* (Available from Focus International, 1-800-843-0305.)

VIDEOS

Best Look Forward. Advice from a makeup artist and hairdresser to women about looking their best during chemotherapy. (Available from Graduate Hospital Cancer Program, Audiovisual Department, 1 Graduate Plaza, Philadelphia, PA 19146, 215-893-2335.)

Heiman, J., and LoPiccolo, J. *Becoming Orgasmic.* A companion book and video self-help program for women who want to be more easily orgasmic. (Available from Focus International, 1-800-843-0305.)

Making It . . . Safe. A Video for heterosexuals and gays that teaches skills in asking for safer sex. (Available from Focus International, 1-800-843-0305.)

A Significant Journey: Breast Cancer Survivors and the Men Who Love Them. How couples communicate about intimacy and sex. (Available from TLC, American Cancer Society, 1-800-850-9445.)

PRODUCTS TO ENHANCE SEX

Mail Order Outlets

Focus International, 1160 East Jericho Turnpike, Huntington, NY 11743, 1-800-843-0305. Offers a variety of education-oriented videotapes about sexuality.

The Good Vibrations Catalogue, 938 Howard St., Suite 101, San Francisco, CA 94103, 1-800-289-8243. Has lubricants, vibrators, and other sex toys. Mail has the return address "Open Enterprises," and your name is not sold to other mailing lists.

The Sexuality Library, 938 Howard St., Suite 101, San Francisco, CA 94103, 1-800-289-8423. Offers a variety of educational (and more entertainment-oriented) books about sexuality; includes feminist ratings of adult videos.

The Xandria Collection, 874 Dubuque Ave., South San Francisco, CA 94080, 1-800-242-2823. Offers lubricants, vibrators, and other products. Mail has the return address "Lawrence Research Group," and your name is not sold to other mailing lists.

Lubricants

These lubricants are available without a prescription:

Astroglide has a thin texture and does not dry out quickly. If it dries out, you can rewet it with water or saliva. Biofilm, Inc., 3121 Scott St., Vista, CA 92083. Call 1-800-325-5695 for a store in your area that carries Astroglide, or try the mail order catalogs under Mail Order Outlets.

Replens is a vaginal moisturizer, designed to be used three times a week. Columbia Laboratories, Inc., Miami, FL 33169. Available in pharmacies.

Vaginal Dilators

The Good Vibrations Catalogue offers small vibrators called "Smoothies" in a variety of sizes. They also market a series of penis-shaped dildoes made out of silicone or rubber that vary in size. Even the smaller ones may be too thick for a woman with severe vaginismus, however.

Latex vaginal dilator sets are manufactured by Milex Products, 5915 Northwest Highway, Chicago, IL 60631. Available only through a physician's prescription.

INFORMATION NETWORKS

Cancer, General

The American Cancer Society (ACS), National Headquarters, 1599 Clifton Rd., NE, Atlanta, GA 30329-4521, 1-800-ACS-2345. Internet: http://www.cancer.org. The ACS has divisions in every state and local chapters in many cities. Support programs include Reach to Recovery and Renu, for breast

cancer; Man to Man, for prostate cancer; Look Good, Feel Better, for chemotherapy patients; and I Can Cope, for all sites. For your nearest office, look in
the telephone book or call your state division.

The Cancer Information Service of the National Cancer Institute, 1-800-4-
CANCER. Internet: http://cancernet.nci.nih.gov/patient.htm. Provides information on all aspects of cancer.

The National Coalition for Cancer Survivorship (NCCS), 1010 Wayne Ave.,
5th Floor, Silver Spring, MD 20910, 301-650-8868. A national advocacy organization that also has local chapters.

Cancer, Specific Types

Let's Face It, P.O. Box 29972, Bellingham, WA 98228-1972, 360-676-7325 (Director: Betsy Wilson). A national information and support group with a number of local chapters for people who have had cancer that affected their facial
appearance.

Man to Man. A network of local support groups for men with prostate cancer.
For information, contact your nearest American Cancer Society office. Internet:
http://www.cancer.org.

The National Alliance of Breast Cancer Organizations (NABCO), 9 East 37th
St., 10th Floor, New York, NY 10016, 1-800-719-9154. Internet: http://
www.nabco.org. Promotes breast cancer research funding and legislation for
survivors and women at risk. It is a clearinghouse for breast cancer information and publishes an annual Breast Cancer Resource List you can order for a
small shipping and handling fee.

The National Prostate Cancer Coalition, 1300 19th St., NW, Suite 400, Washington, DC 20036. Advocates for prostate cancer research and legislation.

The Prostate Cancer Info Link, Internet: http://www.comed.com/prostate/menu/
support.html. This Web site acts as a clearinghouse of information on prostate
cancer, including newsworthy medical information, opportunities for on-line
communication, and referrals to other advocacy organizations.

United Ostomy Association, Inc., 36 Executive Park, Suite 120, Irvine, CA 92714,
714-660-8624. Provides information and support for people with ostomies; also
has local chapters.

US-TOO, International, Inc., 930 N. York Rd., Suite 50, Hinsdale, IL 60521, 1-
800-80-USTOO, Internet: http://www.ustoo.com/test.html. A national prostate cancer and enlarged prostate survivor support group with local chapters.

Y-ME National Breast Cancer Organization, 212 W. Van Buren St., Chicago, IL
50507. National toll-free hotline, 1-800-221-2141 (9 to 5 Central Standard
Time, Monday through Friday), Internet: http://www.Y-ME.org. Has a national
office and local chapters providing information and support, and publishes the
brochure *For Single Women with Breast Cancer*.

Children of Cancer Survivors

Families of Children with Cancer (FCC). An organization based in Toronto that
offers information and help to families of children with cancer and survivors

of childhood cancer. They can be reached only through their Web site on the Internet: http://www.interlog.com/~fcc/.

Registry for children exposed to cancer treatment during conception and pregnancy: Contact John Mulvihill, M.D., Director, The Cancer Genetics Program of the University of Pittsburgh Medical Center, 1-800-237-4724.

Sexual Counseling

The American Association of Sex Educators, Counselors and Therapists (AASECT), 435 North Michigan Ave., Suite 1717, Chicago, IL 60611, 312-644-0828, Internet: http://www.oralcaress.com/AASECT.html. An organization whose members have at least a minimum amount of training in sex therapy.

The Society for Sex Therapy and Research (SSTAR) (Peter J. Fagan, Ph.D., President), Sexual Behaviors Consultation Unit, 550 North Broadway, Suite 114, Baltimore, MD 21205, 410-955-6318. Has lists of mental health professionals with credentials in sex therapy.

Osteoporosis

The National Osteoporosis Foundation, P.O. Box 96173, Washington, DC 20077-7456, Internet: http://www.nof.org. Has information about preventing and treating osteoporosis.

Infertility

American Society for Reproductive Medicine (ASRM), 1209 Montgomery Highway, Birmingham, AL 35216-2809, 205-978-5000, Internet: http://www.asrm.com. For Society for Reproductive Technology (SART) reports, write ASRM or fax: 205-978-5005, or use Web site.

The Organization of Parents through Surrogacy, 7054 Quito Court, Camarillo, CA 93012, 805-482-1566, Internet: http://www.OPTS.com/. Offers information about surrogate motherhood.

Resolve, 1310 Broadway, Somerville, MA 02144-1731, HelpLine 617-623-0744, Internet: http://www.resolve.org/. National information and support organization for infertility; also sponsors local chapters.

Genetic Testing and Counseling

The Alliance of Genetic Support Groups, 35 Wisconsin Circle, Suite 440, Chevy Chase, MD 20815, 1-800-336-GENE. Has information on support groups for families who share genetic risk for cancer.

The Gene Letter, Internet: http//www.geneletter.org/. This Web site presents a newsletter with information a layperson can understand about important medical, ethical, and psychological issues related to genetics, including genetic testing for cancer risk.

The National Cancer Institute publishes a booklet, *Understanding Gene Testing* (96-3905). Order by calling 1-800-4-CANCER.

The National Center for Genome Resources, 1800 Old Pecos Trail, Santa Fe, NM 87505, 505-982-7840, Internet: http//ncgr.org (click on Genetics and

Public Issues). Up-to-date information on genetics and cancer and on public policy issues.

The National Society of Genetic Counselors, 233 Canterbury Drive, Wallingford, PA 19086, 610-872-7608. Can refer you to a counselor in the Familial Cancer Risk Counseling Alliance.

Adoption

Adoptive Families of America (AFA), 333 Highway 100 North, Minneapolis, MN 55422, 612-535-4829 or 1-800-372-3300, Internet: http://www.adoptivefam.org/index.html. Their resources include a magazine, *Adoptive Families*; a yearly conference for adoption consumers; a booklet, *Adoption: How to Begin*; and a catalog of materials and toys for adopted children.

The American Academy of Adoption Attorneys (AAAA), P.O. Box 33053, Washington, DC 20033-0053. A national association for lawyers involved in adoption.

The North American Council on Adoptable Children (NACAC), 970 Raymond Ave. #106, St. Paul, MN 55114-1149, 612-644-3036. Devotes its resources to children who are waiting for homes and may have special needs.

Gay and Lesbian Health

Gay Men's Health Crisis; Education, 212-807-7517, Internet: http://www.gmhc.org. Provides advocacy and information for men and women with HIV and HIV-related cancer.

The Mary-Helen Mautner Project for Lesbians with Cancer, 1707 L St., NW, Suite 1060, Washington, DC 20036, 202-332-5536. Offers family coordinators in the local area, a list of health care practitioners who are sensitive to women's issues, and information on resources in other cities as part of the National Coalition of Feminist and Lesbian Cancer Projects.

The National Lesbian and Gay Health Association, 1407 S St., NW, Washington, DC 20009, 202-939-7880. Provides health advocacy and health information for gay men and women.

Bibliography

INTRODUCTION

Sex and marital satisfaction

Jacobson, N. S., and Margolin, G. *Marital therapy: Strategies Based on Social Learning and Behavior Exchange Principles*, pp. 13–22. New York: Brunner/Mazel, 1979.

Sex and aging

Brecher, E. M. *Love, Sex, and Aging: A Consumer's Union report*. Mt. Vernon, NY: Consumer's Union, 1984.

HOW TO USE THIS BOOK

Ethnicity and sexual attitudes

Wyatt, G. E. "Identifying stereotypes of Afro-American sexuality and their impact upon sexual behavior." In B. A. Bass, G. E. Wyatt, and G. E. Powell (eds.), *The Afro-American Family: Assessment, Treatment, and Research Issues*, pp. 333–346. New York: Grune & Stratton, 1982.

CHAPTER 1

Sex does not stimulate prostate cancer

Schover, L. R. "Sexual rehabilitation after treatment for prostate cancer." *Cancer* 71 (Suppl.) (1993): 1024–1030.

Sexually transmitted viruses linked to cancer

Karp, J. E., Groopman, J. E., and Broder, S. "Cancer in AIDS." In V. T. DeVita, S. Hellman, and S. A. Rosenberg (eds.), *Cancer: Principles and Practice of Oncology* (4th ed.), pp. 2093–2110. Philadelphia: J. B. Lippincott, 1993.

Divorce not more common after cancer

Schover, L. R., and Montague, D. K. "Supportive care and the quality of life of the cancer patient: Sexual problems." In V. T. DeVita, S. Hellman, and S. A. Rosenberg (eds.), *Cancer: Principles and Practice of Oncology* (5th ed.), pp. 2857–2872. Philadelphia: J. B. Lippincott, 1997.

Rates of depression and cancer

McDaniel, J. S., Musselman, D. L., Porter, M. R., Reed, D. A., and C. B. Nemeroff. "Depression in patients with cancer: Diagnosis, biology, and treatment." *Archives of General Psychiatry* 52 (1995): 89–99.

Gender roles and cancer

Compas, B. E., Worsham, N. L., Epping-Jordan, J., et al. "When mom or dad has cancer: Markers of psychological distress in cancer patients, spouses, and children." *Health Psychology* 13 (1994): 507–515.

Northouse, L. L., and Peters-Golden, H. "Cancer and the family: Strategies to assist spouses." *Seminars in Oncology Nursing* 9 (1993): 74–82.

CHAPTER 2

How often men have sex

Laumann, E. O., Gagnon, J. H., Michael, R. T., and Michaels, S. *The Social Organization of Sexuality: Sexual Practices in the United States*, pp. 86–93. Chicago: University of Chicago Press, 1994.

Rates of erection problems with aging

Feldman, A., Goldstein, I., Hatzichristou, G., Krane, R. J., and McKinlay, J. B. "Impotence and its medical and psychosocial correlates: Results of the Massachusetts male aging study." *Journal of Urology* 151 (1994): 54–61.

Hormones and sexual desire

Segraves, R. T. "Hormones and libido." In S. R. Leiblum and R. C. Rosen (eds.), *Sexual Desire Disorders*, pp. 271–312. New York: Guilford Publications, 1988.

Mechanisms of erection

Melman, A. "Neural and vascular control of erection." In R. C. Rosen and S. R. Leiblum (eds.), *Erectile Disorders: Assessment and Treatment*, pp. 55–71. New York: Guilford Publications, 1992.

Mechanisms of male orgasm

Recker, F., and Tscholl, R. "Monitoring of emission as direct intraoperative control for nerve-sparing retroperitoneal lymphadenectomy." *Journal of Urology* 150 (1993): 1360–1364.

Sex and male aging

Schiavi, R. C., Schreiner-Engel, P., Mandeli, J., Schanzer, H., and Cohen, E. "Healthy aging and male sexual function." *American Journal of Psychiatry* 147 (1990): 766–771.

CHAPTER 3

Orgasms and women's age

Morokoff, P. "Determinants of female orgasm." In J. LoPiccolo and L. LoPiccolo (eds.), *Handbook of Sex Therapy*, pp. 167–174. New York: Plenum Press, 1978.

Androgens and women's sexual desire

Sherwin, B. B. "A comparative analysis of the role of androgen in human male and female sexual behavior: Behavioral specificity, critical thresholds, and sensitivity." *Psychobiology* 16 (1988): 416–425.

Evolution of women's orgasms

Glantz, K., and Pearce, J. K. *Exiles from Eden: Psychotherapy from an Evolutionary Perspective*, p. 106. New York: W. W. Norton, 1989.

Baker, R. R., and Bellis, M. A. *Human Sperm Competition: Copulation, Masturbation, and Infidelity*, pp. 229–249. London: Chapman & Hall, 1995.

Female ejaculation

Ladas, A. K., Whipple, B., and Perry, J. D. *The G Spot and Other Recent Discoveries about Human Sexuality.* New York: Holt, Rinehart & Winston, 1982.

Depression not increased at menopause

McKinlay, J. B., McKinlay, S. M., and Brambilla, D. J. "Health status and utilization behavior associated with menopause." *American Journal of Epidemiology* 125 (1987): 110–121.

Benefits of estrogen replacement

Grady, D., Rubin, S. M., Petitti, D. B., et al. "Hormone therapy to prevent disease and prolong life in postmenopausal women." *Archives of Internal Medicine* 15 (1992): 1016–1020.

Risk of breast cancer with estrogen replacement

Colditz, G. A., Hankinson, S. E., Hunter, D. J., et al. "The use of estrogens and progestins and the risk of breast cancer in postmenopausal women." *New England Journal of Medicine* 332 (1995): 1589–1596.

Estrogen may protect against colon cancer

Calle, E. E., Miracle-McMahill, H., Thun, M. J., and Heath, C. W. "Estrogen replacement therapy and risk of fatal colon cancer in a prospective cohort of postmenopausal women." *Journal of the National Cancer Institute* 87 (1995): 517–523.

CHAPTER 5

Lifetime rates of masturbation

Laumann, E. O., Gagnon, J. H., Michael, R. T., and Michaels, S. *The Social Organization of Sexuality: Sexual Practices in the United States*, pp. 80–86. Chicago: University of Chicago Press, 1994.

Masters and Johnson

Masters, W. H., and Johnson, V. E. *Human Sexual Inadequacy*. Boston: Little, Brown, 1970.

CHAPTER 6

Safer sex

Andrist, L. C. "Taking a sexual history and educating clients about safe sex." *Nursing Clinics of North America* 23 (1988): 959–973.

Chemotherapy drugs in semen

Sherins, R. J. "Gonadal dysfunction." In V. T. DeVita, S. Hellman, and S. A. Rosenberg (eds.), *Cancer: Principles and Practice of Oncology* (4th ed.), pp. 2395–2406. Philadelphia: J. B. Lippincott, 1993.

Times to avoid pregnancy

Mulvihill, J. J. "Genetic counseling of the cancer patient." In V. T. DeVita, S. Hellman, and S. A. Rosenberg (eds.), *Cancer: Principles and Practice of Oncology* (4th ed.), pp. 2529–2537. Philadelphia: J. B. Lippincott, 1993.

Sherins, R. J. "Gonadal dysfunction." In V. T. DeVita, S. Hellman, and S. A. Rosenberg (eds.), *Cancer: Principles and Practice of Oncology* (4th ed.), pp. 2395–2406. Philadelphia: J. B. Lippincott, 1993.

Sexually transmitted diseases and cancer

Karp, J. E., Groopman, J. E., and Broder, S. "Cancer in AIDS." In V. T. DeVita, S. Hellman, and S. A. Rosenberg (eds.), *Cancer: Principles and Practice of Oncology* (4th ed.), pp. 2093–2110. Philadelphia: J. B. Lippincott, 1993.

CHAPTER 8

Medications and sexual desire

Segraves, R. T. "Drugs and desire." In S. R. Leiblum and R. D. Rosen (eds.), *Sexual Desire Disorders*, pp. 313–347. New York: Guilford Publications, 1988.

Hormones and sexual desire after cancer treatment

Schover, L. R., and Montague, D. K. "Supportive care and the quality of life of the cancer patient: Sexual problems." In V. T. DeVita, S. Hellman, and S. A. Rosenberg (eds.), *Cancer: Principles and Practice of Oncology* (5th ed.), pp. 2857–2872. Philadelphia: J. B. Lippincott, 1997.

Premature menopause and sexual desire

Kaplan, H. S., and Owett, T. "The female androgen deficiency syndrome." *Journal of Sex and Marital Therapy* 19 (1993): 3–24.

CHAPTER 9

Medications and sexual desire

Segraves, R. T. "Hormones and libido." In S. R. Leiblum and R. C. Rosen (eds.), *Sexual Desire Disorders*, pp. 271–312. New York: Guilford Publications, 1988.

Mechanisms of erection

Melman, A. "Neural and vascular control of erection." In R. C. Rosen and S. R. Leiblum (eds.), *Erectile Disorders: Assessment and Treatment*, pp. 55–71. New York: Guilford Publications, 1992.

Yocon and antidepressant side effects

Bartlik, B. D., Kaplan, P., and Kaplan, H. S. "Psychostimulants apparently reverse sexual dysfunction secondary to selective serotonin re-uptake inhibitors." *Journal of Sex and Marital Therapy* 21 (1995): 264–271.

Testosterone replacement for women

Kaplan, H. S., and Owett, T. "The female androgen deficiency syndrome." *Journal of Sex and Marital Therapy* 19 (1993): 3–24.

High androgens may increase risk of breast cancer

Berrino, F., Muti, P., Micheli, A., et al. "Serum sex hormone levels after menopause and subsequent breast cancer." *Journal of the National Cancer Institute* 88 (1996): 291–296.

Inskip, P. D. "Pelvic radiotherapy, sex hormones, and breast cancer." *Cancer Causes and Control* 5 (1994): 471–478.

Zumoff, B. "Hormonal profiles in women with breast cancer." *Obstetrics and Gynecology Clinics of North America* 21 (1994): 751–772.

Variety in married couples' sex lives

Laumann, E. O., Gagnon, J. H., Michael, R. T., and Michaels, S. *The Social Organization of Sexuality: Sexual Practices in the United States*, pp. 96–111. Chicago: University of Chicago Press, 1994.

CHAPTER 10

Hormones and erections

Segraves, R. T. "Hormones and libido." In S. R. Leiblum and R. C. Rosen (eds.), *Sexual Desire Disorders,* pp. 271–312. New York: Guilford Publications, 1988.

Medications interfering with erection

Segraves, R. T., and Segraves, K. B. "Aging and drug effects on male sexuality." In R. C. Rosen and S. R. Leiblum (eds.), *Erectile Disorders: Assessment and Treatment,* pp. 96–138. New York: Guilford Publications, 1992.

Radical prostatectomy and erections

Schover, L. R. "Sexual rehabilitation after treatment for prostate cancer." *Cancer* 71 (Suppl. 3) (1993): 1024–1030.

Walsh, P. C., and Schlegel, P. N. "Radical pelvic surgery with preservation of sexual function." *Annals of Surgery* 391 (1988): 208–216.

Radiation therapy, chemotherapy, and erection problems

Schover, L. R., and Montague, D. K. "Supportive care and the quality of life of the cancer patient: Sexual problems." In V. T. DeVita, S. Hellman, and S. A. Rosenberg (eds.), *Cancer: Principles and Practice of Oncology* (5th ed.), pp. 2857–2872. Philadelphia: J. B. Lippincott, 1997.

Problems after radiotherapy for testicular cancer

Nijman, J. M. "Some aspects of sexual and gonadal function in patients with nonseminomatous germ-cell tumor of the testis." Ph.D. diss. Groningen, Netherlands: Drukkerij Van Denderen BV, 1987.

Schover, L. R., Gonzales, M., and von Eschenbach, A. C. "Sexual and marital relationships after radiotherapy for seminoma." *Urology* 27 (1986): 117–123.

Schover, L. R., and von Eschenbach, A. C. "Sexual and marital relationships after treatment for nonseminomatous testicular cancer." *Urology* 25 (1985): 251–255.

CHAPTER 11

Diagnostic tests for erectile dysfunction

Schiavi, R. C. "Laboratory methods for evaluating erectile dysfunction." In R. C. Rosen and S. R. Leiblum (eds.), *Erectile Disorders: Assessment and Treatment,* pp. 141–170. New York: Guilford Publications, 1992.

Vacuum devices and penile injections to treat erection problems

Althof, S. E., and Turner, L. A. "Self-injection therapy and external vacuum devices in the treatment of erectile dysfunction: Methods and outcome." In R. C. Rosen and S. R. Leiblum (eds.), *Erectile Disorders: Assessment and Treatment,* pp. 283–309. New York: Guilford Publications, 1992.

Tables in Chapter 11 modified from: Schover, L. R. "Choosing a Treatment for an Erection Problem: A Guide for Patients." Patient education booklet, Center for Sexual Function, Cleveland Clinic Foundation, Cleveland, 1994.

Penile injections to help recovery of erections after cancer surgery

Montrosi, F., Guazzoni, G., Barbieri, L., Consonni, P., Ferini, S., and Rigatti, P. "Abstract: Recovery of spontaneous erectile function after nerve-sparing radical prostatectomy with and without early intracavernous injections of prostaglandin E_1: Results of a prospective randomized trial." *Journal of Urology* 155 (Suppl.) (1996): 628.

Moreland, R. B., Traish, A., McMillin, M. A., Smith, B., Golstein, I., and de Tejada, I. S. "PGE1 suppresses the induction of collagen synthesis by transforming growth factor-ß₁ in human corpus cavernosum smooth muscle." *Journal of Urology* 153 (1995): 826–831.

Pain with prostaglandin injections after cancer surgery

Lakin, M. M., Chen, R. N., Llorens, S. A., Klein, E. A., and Montague, D. K. "Abstract: Prostaglandin E_1 injection therapy for post-prostatectomy impotence: An outcome analysis." *Journal of Urology* 155 (Suppl.) (1996): 639.

Using penile prosthesis surgery to treat erection problems

Melman, A., and Tiefer, L. "Surgery for erectile disorders: Operative procedures and psychological issues." In R. C. Rosen and S. R. Leiblum (eds.), *Erectile Disorders: Assessment and Treatment*, pp. 255–282. New York: Guilford Publications, 1992.

Schover, L. R. "Sex therapy for the penile prosthesis recipient." *Urologic Clinics of North America* 16 (1989): 91–98.

Special issues in using a penile prosthesis after cancer treatment

Scott, F. B., Light, J. K., and Fishman, I. J. "Treatment of impotency caused by cancer therapy: The inflatable penile prosthesis." *Cancer Bulletin* 34 (1992): 33–43.

Sex therapy for erection problems

LoPiccolo, J. "Postmodern sex therapy for erectile failure." In R. C. Rosen and S. R. Leiblum (eds.), *Erectile Disorders: Assessment and Treatment*, pp. 171–197. New York: Guilford Publications, 1992.

CHAPTER 12

Orgasm problems in cancer sex rehabilitation clinic

Schover, L. R. "Sexual rehabilitation after treatment for prostate cancer." *Cancer* 71 (Suppl.) (1993): 1024–1030.

Orgasm problems and antidepressants

Segraves, R. T. "Antidepressant induced orgasm disorder." *Journal of Sex and Marital Therapy* 21 (1995): 192–201.

Dry orgasms after cancer treatment

Schover, L. R., and Montague, D. K. "Supportive care and the quality of life of the cancer patient: Sexual problems." In V. T. DeVita, S. Hellman, and S. A. Rosenberg (eds.), *Cancer: Principles and Practice of Oncology* (5th ed.), pp. 2857–2872. Philadelphia: J. B. Lippincott, 1997.

Sensation with dry orgasm

Schover, L. R., Evans, R. B., and von Eschenbach, A. C. "Sexual rehabilitation and male radical cystectomy." *Journal of Urology* 136 (1986): 1015–1017.

CHAPTER 13

Vaginal effects of radiotherapy

Abitbol, M. M., and Davenport, J. H. "The irradiated vagina." *Obstetrics and Gynecology* 249 (1974): 44–47.

Vaginal effect of bone marrow transplants

Schubert, M. A., Ullivan, K. M., Schubert, M. M., et al. "Gynecologic abnormalities following allogeneic bone marrow transplantation." *Bone Marrow Transplantation* 5 (1990): 425.

Genital pain in men

Schover, L. R. "Psychological factors in men with genital pain." *Cleveland Clinic Journal of Medicine* 57 (1990): 697–700.

CHAPTER 14

Use of Replens for vaginal dryness

Nachtigall, L. E. "Comparative study: Replens versus local estrogen in menopausal women." *Fertility and Sterility* 61 (1994): 178–181.

CHAPTER 16

Tests for male infertility

Hill, L. K., and Lipshultz, L. I. "Routine evaluation of the subfertile male." In E. A. Tanagho, T. F. Lue, and R. D. McClure (eds.), *Contemporary Manage-*

ment of Impotence and Infertility, pp. 213–221. Baltimore, MD: Williams and Wilkins, 1988.

Ovarian reserve and tests for ovulation

American Society for Reproductive Medicine. *Fertility after Cancer Treatment: A Guide for Patients*. Birmingham, AL: American Society for Reproductive Medicine, 1995.

American Society for Reproductive Medicine. *Guideline for Practice: Age-Related Infertility*. Birmingham, AL: American Society for Reproductive Medicine, 1995.

CHAPTER 17

Radiation therapy, chemotherapy, and spermatogenesis

Nicholson, H. S., and Byrne, J. "Fertility and pregnancy after treatment for cancer during childhood or adolescence." *Cancer* 71 (Suppl. 10) (1993): 3392–3399.

Sherins, R. J. "Gonadal dysfunction." In V. T. DeVita, S. Hellman, and S. A. Rosenberg (eds.), *Cancer: Principles and Practice of Oncology* (4th ed.), pp. 2395–2406. Philadelphia: J. B. Lippincott, 1993.

Young men who refuse sperm banking

Cella, D., and Najavits, L. "Letter to the editor: Denial of infertility in patients with Hodgkin's disease." *Psychosomatics* 27 (1986): 71.

Sperm banking before cancer treatment

Agarwal, A., Shekarriz, M., Sidhu, R. S., and Thomas, A. J. Jr. "Value of clinical diagnosis in predicting the quality of cryopreserved sperm from cancer patients." *Journal of Urology* 155 (1996): 934–938.

Agarwal, A., Sidhu, R. K., Shekarriz, M., and Thomas, A. J. Jr. "Optimum abstinence time for cryopreservation of semen in cancer patients." *Journal of Urology* 154 (1995): 86–88.

Agarwal, A., Tolentino, M. V. Jr., Sidhu, R. S., et al. "Effect of cryopreservation on semen quality in patients with testicular cancer." *Urology* 46 (1995): 382–389.

Cleveland Clinic Foundation. *Therapeutic Sperm Banking: An Option for Preserving Male Fertility*. Cleveland, OH: Cleveland Clinic Foundation, 1993.

Practice of sperm banking in the United States

Baker, D. J., and Paterson, M. A. "Marketed sperm: Use and regulation in the United States." *Fertility and Sterility* 63 (1995): 947–952.

CHAPTER 18

Modified node dissection for testicular cancer

Recker, F., and Tscholl, R. "Monitoring of emission as direct intraoperative control for nerve-sparing retroperitoneal lymphadenectomy." *Journal of Urology* 150 (1993): 1360–1364.

Surveillance for testicular cancer

Einhorn, L. H., Richie, J. P., and Shipley, W. U. "Cancer of the testis." In V. T. DeVita, S. Hellman, and S. A. Rosenberg (eds.), *Cancer: Principles and Practice of Oncology* (4th ed.), pp. 1126–1151. Philadelphia: J. B. Lippincott, 1993.

Techniques to achieve pregnancy with men with dry orgasm

Hakim, L. S., Lobel, S. M., and Oates, R. D. "The achievement of pregnancies using assisted reproductive technologies for male factor infertility after retroperitoneal lymph node dissection for testicular carcinoma." *Fertility and Sterility* 64 (1995): 1141–1146.

Intracytoplasmic sperm injection

Oehninger, S., Veeck, L., Lanzendorf, S., et al. "Intracytoplasmic sperm injection: Achievement of high pregnancy rates in couples with severe male factor infertility is dependent primarily upon female and not male factors." *Fertility and Sterility* 64 (1995): 977–981.

Palermo, G. D., Cohen, J., Alikani, M., Adler, A., and Rosenwaks, Z. "Intracytoplasmic sperm injection: A novel treatment for all forms of male factor infertility." *Fertility and Sterility* 63 (1995): 1231–1240.

SART registry for 1994

Society for Assisted Reproductive Technology, American Society for Reproductive Medicine. "Assisted reproductive technology in the United States and Canada: 1994 results generated from the American Society for Reproductive Medicine/Society for Assisted Reproductive Technology Registery." *Fertility and Sterility* 66 (1996): 697–705.

CHAPTER 19

Cancer treatments and female fertility

Nicholson, H. S., and Byrne, J. "Fertility and pregnancy after treatment for cancer during childhood or adolescence." *Cancer* 71 (Suppl. 10) (1993): 3392–3399.

Sherins, R. J. "Gonadal dysfunction." In V. T. DeVita, S. Hellman, and S. A. Rosenberg (eds.), *Cancer: Principles and Practice of Oncology* (4th ed.), pp. 2395–2406. Philadelphia: J. B. Lippincott, 1993.

American Society for Reproductive Medicine. *Fertility after Cancer Treatment: A Guide for Patients.* Birmingham, AL: American Society for Reproductive Medicine, 1995.

Moving the ovaries to avoid radiation damage

Feeney, D. D., Moore, D. H., Look, K. Y., Stehman, F. B., and Sutton, G. P. "The fate of the ovaries after radical hysterectomy and ovarian transposition." *Gynecological Oncology* 56 (1995): 3–8.

Chemotherapy and ovarian damage

Bines, J., Oleske, D. M., and Cobleigh, M. A. "Ovarian function in premenopausal women treated with adjuvant chemotherapy for breast cancer." *Journal of Clinical Oncology* 14 (1996): 1718–1729.

Preserving ovarian function

Redman, J. R., and Bajorunas, D. R. "Suppression of germ cell proliferation to prevent gonadal toxicity associated with cancer treatment." Proceedings of the Workshop on Psychosexual and Reproductive Issues Affecting Patients with Cancer, pp. 90–94. American Cancer Society, January 1987 San Antonio, TX.

Blumenfeld, Z., Avivi, R., Linn, S., Epelbaum, R., Ben-Shahar, M., and Haim, N. "Prevention of irreversible chemotherapy-induced ovarian damage in young women with lymphoma by a gonadotropin-releasing hormone agonist in parallel to chemotherapy." *Human Reproduction* 11 (1996): 1620–1626.

Embryo banking

el Hussein, E., and Tan, S. L. "Successful in vitro fertilization and embryo transfer after treatment of invasive carcinoma of the breast." *Fertility and Sterility* 58 (1992): 194–196.

Pregnancies with cryopreserved oocytes

Toth, T. L., Baka, S. G., Veeck, L. L., Jones, H. W. Jr., Muasher, S., and Lazendorf, S. E. "Fertilization and in vitro development of cryopreserved human prophase 1 oocytes." *Fertility and Sterility* 61 (1994): 891–894.

Toth, T. L., Hassen, W. A., Lazendorf, S. E., Hansen, K., Sandow, B. A., Hodgen, G. D., and Veeck, L. L. "Cryopreservation of human prophase I oocytes collected from unstimulated follicles." *Fertility and Sterility* 61 (1994): 1077–1082.

Ovary banking

Genetics & IVF Institute (Fairfax, VA). Advertisement. *New York Times Magazine,* March 10, 1996, 90.

Gosden, R. G., Baird, D. T., Wade, J. C., and Webb, R. "Restoration of fertility to oophorectomized sheep by ovarian autografts stored at −196 degrees C." *Human Reproduction* 9 (1994): 597–603.

American Society for Reproductive Medicine. Press release, April 8, 1996: ASRM Statement on Cryopreservation of Ovarian Tissue for Future Reimplantation in Women Undergoing Cancer Treatment.

Infertility drugs and ovarian cancer

Bristow, R. D., and Karlan, B. Y. "Ovulation induction, infertility, and ovarian cancer risk." *Fertility and Sterility* 66 (1996): 499–507.

Risch, H. A., Marrett, L. D., and Howe, G. R. "Parity, contraception, infertility, and the risk of epithelial ovarian cancer." *American Journal of Epidemiology* 140 (1994): 585–597.

Rossing, M. A., Daling, J. R., Weiss, N. S., Moore, D. E., and Self, S. G. "Ovarian tumors in a cohort of infertile women." *New England Journal of Medicine* 331 (1994): 771–776.

Venn, A., Watson, L., Lumley, J., Giles, G., King, C., and Healy, D. "Breast and ovarian cancer incidence after infertility and in vitro fertilization." *Lancet* 346 (8981) (1995): 995–1000.

CHAPTER 20

Safety of pregnancy after cancer

Mulvihill, J. J. "Genetic counseling of the cancer patient." In V. T. DeVita, S. Hellman, and S. A. Rosenberg (eds.), *Cancer: Principles and Practice of Oncology* (4th ed.), pp. 2529–2537. Philadelphia: J. B. Lippincott, 1993.

Sherins, R. J. "Gonadal dysfunction." In V. T. DeVita, S. Hellman, and S. A. Rosenberg (eds.), *Cancer: Principles and Practice of Oncology* (4th ed.), pp. 2395–2406. Philadelphia: J. B. Lippincott, 1993.

CHAPTER 21

Birth defects in children of cancer survivors

Mulvihill, J. J. "Genetic counseling of the cancer patient." In V. T. DeVita, S. Hellman, and S. A. Rosenberg (eds.), *Cancer: Principles and Practice of Oncology* (4th ed.), pp. 2529–2537. Philadelphia: J. B. Lippincott, 1993.

Nicholson, H. S., and Byrne, J. "Fertility and pregnancy after treatment for cancer during childhood or adolescence." *Cancer* 71 (Suppl. 10) (1993): 3392–3399.

Sherins, R. J. "Gonadal dysfunction." In V. T. DeVita, S. Hellman, and S. A. Rosenberg (eds.), *Cancer: Principles and Practice of Oncology* (4th ed.), pp. 2395–2406. Philadelphia: J. B. Lippincott, 1993.

Genetic inheritance of cancer

Offit, K., and Brown, K. "Quantitating familial cancer risk: A resource for clinical oncologists." *Journal of Clinical Oncology* 12 (1994): 1724–1736.

Peters, J. A. "Familial cancer risk: Part I: Impact on today's oncology practice." *Journal of Oncology Management* (September/October 1994): 20–30.

Peters, J. A. "Familial cancer risk: Part II: Breast cancer risk counseling and genetic susceptibility testing." *Journal of Oncology Management* (November/December 1994): 18–26.

Wetzel, J. N. "Genetic counseling for familial cancer risk." *Hospital Practice* (February 15, 1996): 57–69.

Legal and ethical risks of genetic testing for cancer

Hubbard, R., and Lewontin, R. C. "Pitfalls of genetic testing." *New England Journal of Medicine* 334 (1996): 1192–1193.

Lerman, C., Rimer, B. K., and Engstrom, P. F. "Cancer risk notification: Psychosocial and ethical implications." *Journal of Clinical Oncology* 9 (1991): 1275–1282.

Genetic testing for children

Wertz, D. C., Fanos, J. H., and Reilly, P. R. "Genetic testing for children and adolescents: Who decides?" *Journal of the American Medical Association* 272 (1994): 875–881.

Preimplantation genetic diagnosis

Gibbons, W. E., Gitlin, S. A., Lanzendorf, S. E., Kaufmann, R. A., Slitnick, R., and Hodgen, G. D. "Preimplantation genetic diagnosis for Tay-Sachs disease: Successful pregnancy after pre-embryo biopsy and gene amplification by polymerase chain reaction." *Fertility and Sterility* 63 (1995): 723–728.

CHAPTER 22

Third-party reproduction

American Society for Reproductive Medicine. *Third-Party Reproduction: A Guide for Parents*. Birmingham, AL: American Society for Reproductive Medicine, 1996.

Donor insemination in the United States

Baker, D. J., and Paterson, M. A. "Marketed sperm: Use and regulation in the United States." *Fertility and Sterility* 63 (1995): 947–952.

Study of children born from donor insemination

Golombok, S., Cook, R., Bish, A., and Murray, C. "Families created by the new reproductive technologies: Quality of parenting and social and emotional development of the children." *Child Development* 66 (1995): 285–298.

Motivations of gamete donors

Schover, L. R., Rothmann, S., and Collins, R. L. "The personality and motivation of semen donors: A comparison with oocyte donors." *Human Reproduction* 7 (1992): 575–579.

Statistics on oocyte donation and surrogacy in 1994

Society for Assisted Reproductive Technology/American Society for Reproductive Medicine. "Assisted reproductive technology in the United States and Canada: 1994 results generated from the American Society for Reproductive Medicine/Society for Assisted Reproductive Technology Registry." *Fertility and Sterility* 66 (1996): 697–705.

Pregnancy with egg donation after cancer

Lee, S., Ghalie, R., Kaizer, H., and Sauer, M. V. "Successful pregnancy in a bone marrow transplant recipient following oocyte donation." *Journal of Assisted Reproduction and Genetics* 12 (1995): 294–296.

Ethical and legal issues with third-party reproduction

Holder, A. R. "Legal and ethical issues in assisted reproductive technology." *Infertility and Reproductive Medicine Clinics of North America* 4 (1993): 597–614.

Telling a child about gamete donation

Cook, R., Golombok, S., Bish, A., and Murray, C. "Disclosure of donor insemination: Parental attitudes." *American Journal of Orthopsychiatry* 65 (1995): 549–559.

Klock, S. C., Jacob, M. C., and Maier, D. "A prospective study of donor insemination recipients: Secrecy, privacy, and disclosure." *Fertility and Sterility* 62 (1994): 477–484.

Schover, L. R., Collins, R. L., and Richards, S. "Psychological aspects of donor insemination: Evaluation and follow-up of recipient couples." *Fertility and Sterility* 57 (1992): 583–590.

CHAPTER 23

Statistics on breast cancer

American Cancer Society. *Cancer Facts & Figures—1995.* Atlanta, GA: American Cancer Society, 1995.

Two studies of mastectomy in community samples

Psychological Aspects of Breast Cancer Study Group. "Psychological response to mastectomy: A prospective comparison study." *Cancer* 59 (1987): 189–196.

Vinokur, A. D., Threatt, B. A., Caplan, R. D., and Zimmerman, B. L. "Physical and psychosocial functioning and adjustment to breast cancer: Long-term follow-up of a screening population." *Cancer* 63 (1989): 394–405.

Body image with a breast prosthesis

Reaby, L. L., and Hort, L. K. "Postmastectomy attitudes in women who wear external breast prostheses compared to those who have undergone breast re-constructions." *Journal of Behavioral Medicine* 18 (1995): 55–67.

Overall adjustment to breast cancer

Schag, C. A. C., Ganz, P. A., Polinsky, M. L., Fred, C., Hirji, K., and Petersen, L. "Characteristics of women at risk for psychosocial distress in the year after breast cancer." *Journal of Clinical Oncology* 11 (1993): 783–793.

Schover, L. R. "Sexuality and body image in younger women with breast cancer." (monograph). *Journal of the National Cancer Institute* 16 (1994): 177–182.

Studies comparing mastectomy, lumpectomy, and reconstruction

Schover, L. R., Yetman, R. J., Tuason, L. J., Meisler, E., Esselstyn, C. B., Hermann, R. E., Grundfest-Broniatowski, S., and Dowden, R. V. "Comparison of partial mastectomy with breast reconstruction on psychosocial adjustment, body image, and sexuality." *Cancer* 75 (1995): 54–64.

The breast implant controversy

Angell, M. *Science on Trial: The Clash of Medical Evidence and the Law in the Breast Implant Case*. New York: W. W. Norton, 1996.

The M. D. Anderson study

Schusterman, M. A., Kroll, S. S., Reece, G. P., et al. "Incidence of autoimmune disease in patients after breast reconstruction with silicone gel implants versus autogenous tissue: A preliminary report." *Annals of Plastic Surgery* 31 (1993): 1–6.

The Mayo Clinic study

Gabriel, S. E., O'Fallon, W. M., Kurland, L. T., Beard, C. M., Woods, J. E., and Melton, L. J. "Risk of connective-tissue diseases and other disorders after breast implantation." *New England Journal of Medicine* 330 (1994): 1697–1702.

The Harvard study

Sanchez-Guerrero, J., Colditz, G. A., Karlson, E. W., et al. "Silicone breast implants and the risk of connective-tissue diseases and symptoms." *New England Journal of Medicine* 332 (1995): 1666–1670.

Overlap of implant syndrome with chronic fatigue and fibromyalgia

Calabrese, L. H., Davis, M. E., and Wilke, W. S. "Chronic fatigue syndrome and a disorder resembling Sjogren's Syndrome: A preliminary report." *Clinical Infectious Diseases* 18 (Suppl. 1) (1994): S28–S31.

Chow, H. W., Calabrese, L. H., Wilke, W. S., and Cash, J. M. "Is silicone-associated illness really chronic fatigue syndrome?" *Arthritis and Rheumatism* 38 (1995): S264.

Fenske, T. K., Davis, P., and Aaron, S. L. "Human adjuvant disease revisited: A review of eleven post-augmentation mammoplasty patients." *Clinical and Experimental Rheumatology* 12 (1994): 477–481.

Prophylactic mastectomy for breast cancer risk

Hoskins, K. F., Stopfer, J. E., Calzone, K. A., Merajver, S. D., Rebbeck, T. R., Garber, J. E., and Weber, B. L. "Assessment and counseling for women with a family history of breast cancer: A guide for clinicians." *Journal of the American Medical Association* 273 (1995): 577–585.

King, M. C., Rowell, S., and Love, S. M. "Inherited breast and ovarian cancer: What are the risks? What are the choices?" *Journal of the American Medical Association* 269 (1993): 1975–1980.

Chemotherapy and long-term side effects

Bines, J., Oleske, D. M., and Cobleigh, M. A. "Ovarian function in premenopausal women treated with adjuvant chemotherapy for breast cancer." *Journal of Clinical Oncology* 14 (1996): 1718–1729.

Chemotherapy and premature menopause

Dnistrian, A. M., Schwartx, M. K., Fracchia, A. A., et al. "Endocrine consequences of CMF adjuvant therapy in premenopausal and postmenopausal breast cancer patients." *Cancer* 51 (1983): 803–807.

Survey of women four years after treatment

Schover, L. R., Yetman, R. J., Tuason, L. J., Meisler, E., Esselstyn, C. B., Hermann, R. E., Grundfest-Broniatowski, S., and Dowden, R. V. "Comparison of partial mastectomy with breast reconstruction on psychosocial adjustment, body image, and sexuality." *Cancer* 75 (1995): 54–64.

Chemotherapy and sexual function

Young-McCaughan, S. "Sexual functioning in women with breast cancer after treatment with adjuvant therapy." *Cancer Nursing* 19 (1996): 308–319.

Effectiveness of chemotherapy

Collichio, F., and Pandya, K. "Amenorrhea following chemotherapy for breast cancer: Effect on disease-free survival." *Oncology* 12 (1994): 45–52.

Overmoyer, B. A. "Chemotherapy in the management of breast cancer." *Cleveland Clinic Journal of Medicine* 62 (1995): 36–50.

Impact of tamoxifen on hormonal status

Jaiyesimi, I. A., Buzdar, A. U., Decker, D. A., and Hortobagyi, G. N. "Use of tamoxifen for breast cancer: Twenty-eight years later." *Journal of Clinical Oncology* 13 (1995): 513–529.

Lonning, P. E., Johannessen, D. C., Lien, E. A., et al. "Influence of tamoxifen on sex hormones, gonadotrophins, and sex hormone binding globulin in postmenopausal breast cancer patients." *Journal of Steroid Biochemistry and Molecular Biology* 52 (1995): 491–496.

Tamoxifen and depression

Cathcart, C., Pumroy, S., Peters, G., Knox, S., and Cheek, H. "Frequency, severity, and management of tamoxifen-induced depression in women with node negative breast cancer" (Abstract 112). *Proceedings of The American Society of Clinical Oncology* 12 (1993): 78.

Tamoxifen and sexual desire

National Surgical Adjuvant Breast and Bowel Project (NSABBP). *Handbook: A clinical trial to determine the worth of tamoxifen for preventing breast cancer:* Protocol P-1, Protocol Revision Record, August 13, 1992.

The safety of estrogen replacement after breast cancer

Cobleigh, M. A., Berris, R. F., Bush, T., et al. "Estrogen replacement therapy in breast cancer survivors: A time for change." *Journal of the American Medical Association* 540 (1994): 272–276.

Therialt, R. L., and Sellin, R. V. "Estrogen-replacement therapy in younger women with breast cancer." *Monographs: Journal of the National Cancer Institute* 16 (1994): 149–152.

Impact of tamoxifen

DiSaia, P. J. "Hormone replacement therapy for breast cancer survivors: Facts vs. fears." *International Urogynecology Journal* 6 (1995): 125–129.

DiSaia, P. J., Grosen, E. A., Kurosaki, T., Gildea, M., Cowan, B., and Anton-Culver, H. "Hormone replacement therapy in breast cancer survivors: A cohort study." *American Journal of Obstetrics and Gynecology* 174 (1996): 1494–1498.

Breast cancer and pregnancy

Baron, R. H. "Dispelling the myths of pregnancy-associated breast cancer." *Oncology Nursing Forum* 21 (1994): 507–512.

Dow, K. H. "Having children after breast cancer." *Cancer Practice* 2 (1994): 407–413.

Transient breast cancer risk with first pregnancy

Colditz, G. A., Rosner, B. A., and Speizer, F. E. "Risk factors for breast cancer according to family history of breast cancer." *Journal of the National Cancer Institute* 88 (1996): 365–371.

Lambe, M., Chung-Cheng, H., Trichopoulos, D., Ekbom, A., Pavia, M., and Adami, H. O. "Transient increase in the risk of breast cancer after giving birth." *New England Journal of Medicine* 331 (1994): 5–9.

Pregnancy and prognosis in women under 30

Guinee, V. F., Olsson, H., Moller, T., et al. "Effect of pregnancy on prognosis for young women with breast cancer." *Lancet* 343 (1994): 1587–1589.

Reassuring study of pregnancy after breast cancer

von Schoultz, E., Johansson, H., Wilking, N., and Rutqvist, L. E. "Influence of prior and subsequent pregnancy on breast cancer prognosis." *Journal of Clinical Oncology* 13 (1995): 430–434.

Breast feeding after breast conservation

Tralins, A. H. "Lactation after conservative breast surgery combined with radiation therapy." *American Journal of Clinical Oncology* 18 (1995): 40–43.

CHAPTER 24

Statistics on prostate cancer

American Cancer Society. *Cancer Facts & Figures—1995*. Atlanta, GA: American Cancer Society, 1995.

Controversy over treating localized prostate cancer

Coffey, D. S. "Prostate cancer: An overview of an increasing dilemma." *Cancer* 71 (Suppl. 3) (1993): 880–886.

Fleming, C., Wasson, J. H., Albertsen, P. C., Barry, M. J., and Wennberg, J. E. "A decision analysis of alternative treatment strategies for clinically localized prostate cancer." *Journal of the American Medical Association* 269 (1993): 2650–2658.

Meyer, S., and Nash, S. C. *Prostate Cancer: Making Survival Decisions*. Chicago: University of Chicago Press, 1994.

Nerve-sparing radical prostatectomy

Walsh, P. C., and Schlegel, P. N. "Radical pelvic surgery with preservation of sexual function." *Annals of Surgery* 391 (1988): 208–216.

Dana Farber study

Talcott, J. A. "Quality of life in early prostate cancer. Do we know enough to treat?" *Hematology-Oncology Clinics of North America* 10 (1996): 691–701.

University of Wisconsin study

Jonler, M., Messing, E. M., Rhodes, P. R., and Bruskewitz, R. C. "Sequelae of radical prostatectomy." *British Journal of Urology* 74 (1994): 352–358.

Managed care surveys

Litwin, M. S. "Health-related quality of life after treatment for localized prostate cancer." *Cancer* 75 (1995): 2000–2003.

Litwin, M. S., Hays, R. D., Fink, A., et al. "Quality-of-life outcomes in men treated for localized prostate cancer." *Journal of the American Medical Association* 273 (1995): 129–135.

Murphy, G. P., Mettlin, C., Menck, H., Winchester, D. P., and Davidson, A. M. "National patterns of prostate cancer treatment by radical prostatectomy: Results of a survey by the American College of Surgeons Commission on Cancer." *Journal of Urology* 152 (1994): 1817–1819.

Risk of sexual problems after prostatectomy versus radiotherapy for prostate cancer

Litwin, M. S., Hays, R. D., Fink, A., et al. "Quality-of-life outcomes in men treated for localized prostate cancer." *Journal of the American Medical Association* 273 (1995): 129–135.

Schover, L. R. "Sexual rehabilitation after treatment for prostate cancer." *Cancer* 71 (Suppl. 3) (1993): 1024–1030.

Schover, L. R., and Montague, D. K. "Supportive care and the quality of life of the cancer patient: Sexual problems." In V. T. DeVita, S. Hellman, and S. A. Rosenberg (eds.), *Cancer: Principles and Practice of Oncology* (5th ed.), pp. 2857–2872. Philadelphia: J. B. Lippincott, 1997.

Sexual function after radioactive implantation

Stock, R. G., Stone, N. N., and Iannuzzi, C. "Sexual potency following interactive ultrasound-guided brachytherapy for prostate cancer." *International Journal of Radiation Oncology, Biology, and Physics* 35: 267–272.

Sexual function after cryosurgery for prostate cancer

Klein, E. A. "An update on prostate cancer." *Cleveland Clinic Journal of Medicine* 52 (1995): 325–338.

Improved quality of life with delayed hormonal therapy

Herr, H. W., Kornblith, A. B., and Ofman, U. "A comparison of quality of life of patients with metastatic prostate cancer who received or did not receive hormonal therapy." *Cancer* 71 (Suppl. 3) (1993): 1143–1150.

Androgen-blocking drugs and sexual function

Tyrrell, C. J. "Tolerability and quality of life aspects with the anti-androgen Casodex (ICI 176,334) as monotherapy for prostate cancer." *European Urology* 26 (Suppl.) (1994): 15–19.

Sexual impact of new drug combination

Fleshner, N. E., and Trachtenberg, J. "Treatment of advanced prostate cancer with the combination of finasteride plus flutamide: Early results." *European Urology* 24 (Suppl.) (1993): 106–112.

Finasteride and sexual dysfunction

Gormley, G. J., Stoner, E., Bruskewitz, R. C., et al. "The effect of finasteride in men with benign prostatic hyperplasia. The Finasteride Study Group." *New England Journal of Medicine* 327 (1992): 1185–1191.

Jonler, M., Messing, E. M., Rhodes, P. R., and Bruskewitz, R. C. "Sequelae of radical prostatectomy." *British Journal of Urology* 74 (1994): 352–358.

Stoner, E. "Three-year safety and efficacy data on the use of finasteride in the treatment of benign prostatic hyperplasia." *Urology* 43 (1994): 284–292.

CHAPTER 25

Research study on radical hysterectomy and sex

Schover, L. R., Fife, M., and Gershenson, D. M. "Sexual dysfunction and treatment for early state cervical cancer." *Cancer* 63 (1989): 204–212.

Sex after cancer of the vulva

Andersen, B. L., and Hacker, N. F. "Psychosexual adjustment following vulvar surgery." *Obstetrics and Gynecology* 62 (1983): 457–462.

Weijmar-Schultz, W. C. M., van de Wiel, H. B. M., Bouma, J., Janssens, J., and Littlewood, J. "Psychosexual functioning after the treatment of cancer of the vulva: A longitudinal study." *Cancer* 66 (1990): 402–407.

Sex after radical cystectomy for women

Schover, L. R., and von Eschenbach, A. C. "Sexual function and female radical cystectomy: A case series." *Journal of Urology* 134 (1985): 465–468.

Sex after colorectal cancer surgery or total pelvic exenteration in women

Schover, L. R., and Fife, M. "Sexual counseling with radical pelvic or genital cancer surgery." *Journal of Psychosocial Oncology* 3 (1985): 21–41.

Women who had pelvic exenteration and reconstruction

Ratliff, C. F., Gershenson, D. M., Morris, M., Burke, T. W., Levenback, C., Schover, L. R., Mitchell, M. F., Atkinson, E. N., and Wharton, J. T. "Sexual adjustment in patients undergoing gracilis myocutaneous flap vaginal reconstruction in conjunction with pelvic exenteration." *Cancer* 78 (1996): 2229–2235.

Sex after total penectomy

Witkin, M. H., and Kaplan, H. S. "Sex therapy and penectomy." *Journal of Sex and Marital Therapy* 8 (1982): 209–220.

Sex after radical cystectomy in men

Schover, L. R., Evans, R. B., and von Eschenbach, A. C. "Sexual rehabilitation and male radical cystectomy." *Journal of Urology* 136 (1986): 1015–1017.

Nerve-sparing radical cystectomy

Schoenberg, M. P., Walsh, P. C., Breazeale, D. R., Marshall, F. F., Mostwin, J. L., and Brendler, C. B. "Local recurrence and survival following nerve-sparing radical cystoprostatectomy for bladder cancer: 10-year follow-up." *Journal of Urology* 155 (1996): 490–494.

Sex after colorectal cancer surgery

Enker, W. E. "Potency, cure, and local control in the operative treatment of rectal cancer." *Archives of Surgery* 127 (1992): 1396–1401.

CHAPTER 26

Long-term health and fertility after childhood cancer

Mustieles, C., Munoz, A., Alonso, M., et al. "Male gonadal function after chemotherapy in survivors of childhood malignancy." *Medical and Pediatric Oncology* 24 (1995): 347–351.

Ochs, J., and Mulhern, R. "Long-term sequelae of therapy for childhood acute lymphoblastic leukaemia." *Bailliere's Clinical Haematology* 7 (1994): 365–376.

Strong, L. C. "Genetic implications for long-term survivors of childhood cancer." *Cancer* 71 (1993): 3435–3440.

Health of children of childhood cancer survivors

Nicholson, H. S., and Byrne, J. "Fertility and pregnancy after treatment for cancer during childhood or adolescence." *Cancer* 71 (Suppl. 10) (1993): 3392–3399.

CHAPTER 27

Sexual lifestyles of gay women

Blumstein, P., and Schwartz, P. *American Couples: Money, Work, Sex.* New York: Pocket Books, 1983.

Risk of cancer in gay women

Brownworth, V. A. "The other epidemic: Lesbians and breast cancer." *Out* (February/March 1993).

Rankow, E. J. "Breast and cervical cancer among lesbians." *Women's Health Issues* 5 (1995): 123–129.

Homophobia in health care providers

Rankow, E. J. "Lesbian health issues for the primary care provider." *Journal of Family Practice* 40 (1995): 486–492.

Sexual problems in gay couples

Nichols, M. "Sex therapy with lesbians, gay men, and bisexuals." In S. R. Leiblum and R. C. Rosen, *Principles and Practice of Sex Therapy: Update for the 1990s*, pp. 269–297. New York: Guilford Publications, 1989.

Options for parenting for gay people

Benkov, L. *Reinventing the Family: The Emerging Story of Lesbian and Gay Parents*. New York: Crown Publishers, 1994.

Self-insemination

Wikler, D., and Wikler, N. J. "Turkey-baster babies: The demedicalization of artificial insemination." *The Milbank Quarterly* 69 (1991): 5–40.

Donor insemination for lesbian women

Wedland, C. L., Byrn, F., and Hill, C. "Donor insemination: A comparison of lesbian couples, heterosexual couples, and single women." *Fertility and Sterility* 65 (1996): 764–770.

CHAPTER 28

Health and marital status

Laumann, E. O., Gagnon, J. H., Michael, R. T., and Michaels, S. *The Social Organization of Sexuality: Sexual Practices in the United States*, pp. 225–268, 351–375, 475–508. Chicago: University of Chicago Press, 1994.

Single mothers with breast cancer

Lewis, F. M., Zahlis, E. H., Shands, M. E., Sinsheimer, J. A., and Hammond, M. A. "The functioning of single women with breast cancer and their school-aged children." *Cancer Practice* 4 (1996): 15–24.

Glossary

abdominoperineal resection An operation to remove the colon and rectum to treat colorectal cancer.

adhesions Filmy scar tissue that makes internal organs stick together.

alkylating drugs A class of chemotherapy drugs that is especially likely to damage fertility.

amniocentesis A test for genetic problems in a fetus that uses a needle to obtain fetal cells from the amniotic fluid during the mother's pregnancy.

androgen blockers Medications that block receptors for androgens, preventing the hormones from getting into their target cells.

androgens The group of hormones made in a man's testicles, in a woman's ovaries, and in the adrenal glands in both sexes; includes testosterone.

aphrodisiac A substance that would increase sexual desire.

biopsy Taking a sample of tissue in an area suspicious for cancer so that it can be examined for abnormal cells.

bone marrow transplant Using bone marrow cells either harvested and frozen from the patient's own supply or taken from a matched donor to restore blood cells that have been killed off by chemotherapy or radiation therapy.

cavernous body One of two paired chambers of spongy tissue that form the shaft of the penis and fill with blood during erection.

chemotherapy A variety of toxic medications that are given to patients to kill cancer cells while sparing most healthy cells.

chlamydia A bacterial, sexually transmitted infection that can cause pain with urination and discharge. If untreated it can lead to infertility, especially in women.

chorionic villi sampling (CVS) A test for genetic problems in a fetus that uses a needle to obtain fetal cells from the villi of the placenta during the mother's pregnancy.

colostomy An opening on the abdomen that forms a passageway for stool when the colon and rectum are removed to treat cancer. A colostomy appliance is a faceplate and a bag to contain the stool.

colposcopy A diagnostic test in which the vulvar skin is examined through a special microscope.

cryosurgery Surgery that involves freezing an organ to destroy abnormal tissue.

delirium A mental condition of confusion and disorientation, common in older people after major surgery.

dihydrotestosterone   A stronger form of the hormone testosterone that plays a role in benign overgrowth of the prostate.

ejaculation   The second phase of the male orgasm; includes muscle contractions at the base of the penis that expel the semen in spurts.

electroejaculation   A technique to stimulate ejaculation of semen via an electrical pulse to the anal canal.

emission   The first phase of the male orgasm; includes contraction of the prostate and seminal vesicles to mix up the semen and closure of the valve between the bladder and urethra.

endometrium   The lining of the uterus.

epididymis   An area at the top of the testicle where sperm cells mature and are stored.

estrogen   A hormone produced by the ovaries; regulates the menstrual cycle and promotes vaginal lubrication; also helps bones retain calcium, promotes good cholesterol ratios, and helps maintain good blood flow to the genital area and other organs.

Familial Adenomatous Polyposis (FAP)   A syndrome in which a mutated gene causes formation of colon polyps and, eventually, colon cancer in family members who inherit it.

fibromyalgia   A chronic pain syndrome involving tenderness of the joints and muscles.

fibrosis   A process of scarring in soft tissue; takes place after radiation therapy.

fimbria   Fringelike structures at the opening of each fallopian tube; help guide a ripe egg into the tube.

follicle   A nest of cells that surrounds and nourishes each ripening egg. After ovulation, the follicle continues to produce hormones that regulate the menstrual cycle.

follicle stimulating hormone (FSH)   A hormone produced by the pituitary gland; important in male and female fertility.

gamete   An egg or sperm cell.

gamete intrafallopian transfer (GIFT)   An infertility treatment that involves placing eggs and sperm in the entrance to the fallopian tubes.

genital herpes   A virus that causes painful blisters on the genital area of men or women.

gestational carrier   A woman who carries a pregnancy for an infertile couple who provide the egg and the sperm for the embryo.

graft versus host disease   A side effect of bone marrow transplant from a donor in which the immune system attacks some of the body's own tissues.

Hodgkin's disease   A cancer of the lymph system that often occurs in younger men and women.

hormone therapy   Using hormones to treat hormone-sensitive cancers, such as prostate or breast cancer.

human immunodeficiency virus (HIV)   A virus that destroys the immune system, eventually causing the acquired immunodeficiency syndrome (AIDS). HIV can be transmitted through contact with infected body fluids, such as blood, semen, vaginal secretions, or saliva.

human papilloma virus (HPV)   A sexually transmitted virus that causes warty growths around the genital and anal areas. Warts are usually painless and not dangerous to health, but some varieties of the virus can promote cancer of the cervix, vulva, penis, or anus.

hysterectomy   Surgery to remove the uterus.

ileostomy   An opening created on the abdomen for stool when most of the intestine has been removed.

incontinence   Loss of control over urination or bowel movements.

inflatable penile prosthesis   An artificial pump system surgically placed into the penis and pelvic area to treat an erection problem.

intracytoplasmic sperm injection (ICSI)   An infertility treatment in which a sperm cell is injected into each egg to produce fertilization; a variation of in vitro fertilization.

intrauterine insemination   An infertility treatment in which a concentrated portion of sperm cells is placed directly into the woman's uterus.

in vitro fertilization (IVF)   An infertility treatment that involves stimulating a woman with hormones to produce multiple eggs, harvesting the eggs in a minor surgery, and placing the eggs with sperm cells to fertilize in the laboratory. Fertilized embryos are then replaced in the woman's uterus.

Kaposi's sarcoma   A cancer of the skin and lymph nodes most commonly seen in gay men infected with HIV.

kegels   Exercises to strengthen the pelvic floor muscles.

laparoscopy   A way of performing surgery through a small opening by using a special scope to see and treat the organs inside the body.

laryngectomy   Surgery to remove the larynx, or voice box, for cancer. A tracheostomy is created if the laryngectomy is complete.

leukemia   A cancer affecting the white blood cell system.

Li-Fraumeni syndrome   A type of inherited risk for cancer, including breast cancer, leukemia, brain tumors, and sarcomas; caused by a mutation in the P53 gene.

lumpectomy   A surgery for breast cancer that removes the tumor and some surrounding tissue, but not the entire breast.

luteinizing hormone (LH)   A hormone produced by the pituitary gland; important in male and female fertility.

luteinizing hormone releasing hormone (LHRH)   A hormone made in the hypothalamus of the brain; helps control other hormone production in the body.

luteinizing hormone releasing hormone (LHRH) agonist   A medication that mimics the action of LHRH by fitting into the same cell receptors that the hormone does.

mammogram   An X ray of the breast to diagnose breast cancer.

mantle field   A target area for radiation that includes the shoulders and abdomen; used for Hodgkin's disease.

mastectomy   Surgery to remove a breast.

maturation index   A test that looks at cells from the vaginal lining to see if a woman has high-enough estrogen levels.

menopause   When a woman's menstrual cycles stop because the ovaries stop producing estrogen and progesterone. Menopause normally occurs at about age 51 but can happen prematurely as a result of damage to the ovaries from cancer treatment.

monilia   A vaginal infection caused by a yeast organism.

motility   A measure of the health and liveliness of sperm cells.

nasopharyngeal tumor   A cancer in the nasal cavity or pharynx.

natural cycle IVF   In vitro fertilization that just retrieves whatever eggs ripen naturally, without using hormones to stimulate ovulation.

nerve-sparing surgery   Modifications of cancer surgery, for example, in prostatectomy or lymph node dissection, to avoid damaging nerves important for sexual function or fertility.

neuropathy   Symptoms of damage to a part of the nervous system.

neurotransmitters   Chemicals that carry messages between nerve cells within the nervous system.

oocyte   The egg a woman's ovaries produce.

oophorectomy   Surgery to remove an ovary; *bilateral oophorectomy* involves removing both ovaries.

orchiectomy   Surgery to remove a testicle; *bilateral orchiectomy* involves removing both testicles.

osteoporosis   Thinning of the bones with aging; can lead to fractures and back pain.

ovarian reserve The ovaries' remaining capacity to produce ripe eggs.

ovulation Release of a ripe egg from its follicle on the ovary.

parasympathetic nervous system Part of the involuntary nervous system that controls sexual function.

penectomy Surgery to remove part or all of the penis.

perineal urethrostomy An opening created for the urethra between the scrotum and anus after total penectomy.

Peyronie's disease Scarring of the penile tissues that can produce pain and curvature with erection.

progesterone A hormone produced by the ovaries; helps regulate the menstrual cycle and prepare the uterine lining for pregnancy; can cause depression and irritability.

prolactin A hormone made by the pituitary gland; stimulates milk production in women; too much prolactin interferes with sexual function.

prophylactic surgery An operation to remove an organ that is at risk to develop cancer, but without any cancer diagnosed; as in prophylactic mastectomy or prophylactic oophorectomy.

prostate specific antigen (PSA) A chemical produced in the prostate that can be measured with a blood test; high levels may indicate the presence of prostate cancer.

pubococcygeal (PC) muscle The muscle surrounding the outermost vaginal canal.

rad The unit used to measure the dose of radiation an area receives.

radiation therapy Using radiation aimed at a tumor to kill cancer cells.

radical cystectomy In men, removal of the bladder, prostate, seminal vesicles, and part or all of the urethra; in women, removal of the bladder, urethra, uterus, ovaries, and front vaginal wall; surgery to treat bladder cancer.

radical hysterectomy Removal of the uterus, fallopian tubes, uterine ligaments, and upper vagina to treat cervical cancer.

radical prostatectomy Removal of the prostate and seminal vesicles to treat prostate cancer.

radical surgery Cancer surgery designed to remove all cancer cells, usually including removing an organ that contains cancer along with some healthy tissue all around the edges of the area removed to provide a clean margin of error.

radical vulvectomy Removal of the soft tissue of the vulva, including the clitoris and inner and outer lips; usually also includes a pelvic lymph node dissection.

rapid eye movement (REM) sleep   A stage of sleep in which dreaming, eye movements, reflex erections, and other nervous system activity occur.

receptors   Chemical keyholes on the surface of cells that allow certain substances to enter the cell.

refractory phase   The time after a man's orgasm when he is unable to have a second ejaculation.

retinoblastoma   A cancer of the eye that usually occurs in early childhood and is sometimes hereditary.

retrograde ejaculation   A condition in which semen spurts backward into the bladder during orgasm instead of out through the penis.

retroperitoneal lymphadenectomy   An operation to remove the lymph nodes in the upper abdomen; used to diagnose the spread of testicular cancer.

rhabdomyosarcoma   A connective tissue tumor of childhood.

rheumatoid arthritis   A connective tissue disorder that causes severe joint pain and deformity.

saline   A sterile saltwater solution.

scleroderma   A disease of the connective tissue theorized to be more common in women who have silicone breast implants.

seminoma   A type of testicular cancer arising from the germ cells of the testicle.

sensate focus exercises   A series of touching exercises used in sexual counseling; designed to decrease anxiety about sexual performance.

serotonin reuptake inhibitors   A class of antidepressants that increase the levels of the neurotransmitter serotonin in the brain.

sigmoidectomy   An operation to remove the sigmoid portion of the colon; used to treat colon cancer.

spongy body   The chamber of the penis that surrounds the urethra and fans out to form the glans, or head, of the penis.

stem cells   Cells that produce renewable types of body cells, such as blood cells or sperm cells.

steroids   A family of hormones and medications that includes the androgens and also drugs that suppress the immune system.

surrogate mother   A woman who becomes pregnant through insemination with the sperm of the man in an infertile couple and bears a baby for the couple.

sympathetic nervous system   Part of the involuntary nervous system; controls sexual function.

systemic lupus erythematosus   A connective tissue disorder that can affect the skin or other organ systems.

testosterone   A hormone made in the testicles that is important both for sexual function and fertility. Similar androgen hormones in women also help promote sexual desire.

total pelvic exenteration Removal of the urinary tract, colon, and rectum, plus, in men, the prostate and seminal vesicles, or, in women, the uterus, tubes, ovaries, and vagina. In women, vaginal reconstruction is usually included.

tracheostomy An opening at the neck through the trachea for breathing; created when the larynx is removed in cancer surgery.

transcutaneous electrical stimulation (TENS) unit A machine that uses electrical pulses to reduce pain sensations.

ultrasound study Using sound waves to create an image of an area inside the body.

urethra The tube that connects the bladder to the outside of the body and forms a passageway for urine and, in men, for semen.

urinary tract infections (UTIs) Bacterial infections of the bladder and urethra.

urostomy An opening on the abdomen that forms a passageway for urine when the bladder must be removed to treat bladder cancer. An ostomy appliance is a faceplate and a bag to collect the urine.

vacuum constriction device (VCD) A small pump that can be used to produce an erection by creating a vacuum around the penis.

vaginal aspiration A procedure to retrieve ripe eggs for in vitro fertilization that uses an ultrasound image to guide a needle through the upper vagina and into each follicle.

vaginal dilator A cylindrical object that a woman can place in her vagina to practice muscle relaxation or to stretch the vaginal walls.

vaginismus A tendency to involuntarily contract the muscles surrounding the vaginal entrance, making penetration for intercourse tight and painful.

Wilm's tumor A childhood cancer of the kidney.

zygote intrafallopian transfer (ZIFT) An infertility treatment in which fertilized embryos are placed into the fallopian tubes.

Index